# Rheumatology

## Made Ridiculously Simple

Adam J. Brown, M.D.
Associate Staff
Dept. of Rheumatic & Immunologic Diseases
Cleveland Clinic
Cleveland OH 44195
BROWNA22@ccf.org

Follow on twitter @AdamJBrownMD
Adam J Brown also has a podcast called Rheuminations which discusses interesting medical cases, interviews experts in the field and discusses the history of rheumatology.

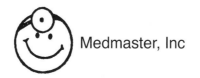

Medmaster, Inc

ISBN #978-1-935660-38-5

*Made in the United States of America*

Published by
MedMaster, Inc.
P.O. Box 640028
Miami, FL 33164

Cover by Richard March

This book is dedicated to my inspiring and supportive family, to my wife Laura Zajdel Brown, M.D. and son Collin Henry Brown. Thank you for your patience when I worked on this book so many nights and weekends.

*Special thanks to:*

*Photographs*
Aviva Hopkins Wolgin, M.D.
American College of Rheumatology

*Illustration Editor*
Stephen Goldberg, M.D.

*The Book Reviewers*
Stephen Goldberg, M.D.
Phyllis Goldenberg

# What Is a Rheumatologist?

A rheumatologist is a physician who specializes in autoimmune and other diseases of the joints and musculoskeletal system.

The immune system's job is recognizing and eliminating infectious diseases, but sometimes the immune system malfunctions and attacks normal organ systems and joints (autoimmunity). The rheumatologist must recognize when this occurs and initiate treatment, which usually involves specialized medications that suppress a component of the immune system. This hopefully will eliminate symptoms and put the disease in remission.

In rheumatoid arthritis, for example, the immune system inappropriately attacks the synovial lining of certain joints, causing joint pain and swelling. Once the disease is recognized, immunosuppressive medications can be initiated and rapidly alleviate the pain and swelling. Rheumatologists usually become very good friends with their patients since we see them often and, hopefully, are keeping them as pain-free as possible.

Besides the broad category of autoimmune disease, rheumatologists also evaluate and treat other causes of joint pain, such as tenosynovitis, osteoarthritis, bursitis, and trigger fingers. Orthopedic surgeons also see patients with joint pains, but a big difference between orthopedic surgeons and rheumatologists is that orthopedic surgeons operate on joints; rheumatologists do not. One of the goals of the rheumatologist is to prevent or slow down joint loss as much as possible, to delay or avoid joint replacement surgery.

I'm clearly biased, but I think rheumatology is the greatest specialty in internal medicine. If you like physiology, problem solving, applying the physical exam and other diagnostic modalities, and administering specialty medications to make a massive difference in a patient's life, then rheumatology may be for you.

Rheumatologists treat a variety of rare diseases that affect multiple organ systems. Unlike many specialties, rheumatology focuses on all the organ systems in the body, as the immune system can affect any of them. Rheumatologists drain fluid from joints and analyze the fluid under a microscope. We look at patients' nails under a microscope, we use bedside ultrasound to evaluate joint pain, and we also collect urine and analyze it under the microscope for evidence of inflammation within the kidney. We look at x-rays of joints as well as MRIs of brains. Also, unlike many specialties, we rely heavily on the physical exam. In a patient with rheumatoid arthritis, for example, the disease may be active, causing pain and swelling in the hands, and the patient's labs may be normal; it's up to the rheumatologist to recognize the symptoms and history as well as the characteristic physical exam findings to diagnose and initiate treatment. Many of the interesting physical exam findings you learn about in medical school are those of rheumatologic diseases!

The job satisfaction for rheumatology is very high because we see some really strange and fascinating diseases, every day is different, and we usually make our patients feel significantly better once the diagnosis is made. Every year we gain a better understanding of the diseases we treat, and we acquire new ways of treating them. Diseases that once had few treatment options now have many options, and diseases that were once debilitating are now less so, allowing patients to live close to normal lives with the aid of medications. If we make the correct diagnosis and initiate the correct treatment, many diseases can be rapidly and successfully treated. If you don't believe this, ask any patient with rheumatoid arthritis or gout.

## Overview of This Book

The aim of this book is to make the nebulous field of rheumatology a little less formidable. Working up a patient with a potential autoimmune disease is not something most medical students and internal medicine residents are comfortable with. Most autoimmune diseases are rare, and they often don't end up in the hospital where you would encounter them. Most medical students and residents become very familiar with heart attacks and heart failure exacerbations without going through a cardiology fellowship because these conditions are common, and you see them in the hospital over and over.

Autoimmune diseases are not only rare, but many have varied presentations with broad differentials, which sometimes makes the diagnosis tricky. This book attempts to break down how to approach a patient with suspected autoimmune disease, how to better understand the disease manifestations, and how to interpret the lab tests and feel comfortable making the diagnosis. One of the most important things you can do for a patient is to recognize when the symptoms are of autoimmune etiology; even if you're not able to put a label to the diagnosis, you can initiate appropriate therapy, dramatically alleviate symptoms, and potentially save a life. Joint pain is a common symptom; one of the goals of this book is to learn to recognize the patterns that are seen when joint pain is caused by an autoimmune process.

It's important to stress that we do not understand why most autoimmune diseases occur. The field of rheumatology is still in its early stages of understanding the pathophysiology of autoimmunity. We also don't understand why certain diseases selectively attack particular organ systems or joints. It's good to know that certain joints are typically involved in rheumatoid arthritis, but we don't know why other joints are not. Why are the metacarpophalangeal joints involved in rheumatoid arthritis but not the distal interphalangeal joints? Why does microscopic polyangiitis attack the lungs and the kidneys but usually spares everything else? The answer is...We don't know! I hope that decreases your stress a little bit. The good news: Even if we don't know what first triggered these diseases, we often do understand the underlying drivers of the diseases once they get started, which has led to monumentally better treatment options.

Rheumatology is a fun field with incredibly strange diseases to diagnose and treat. I hope this book sparks some interest in the field and allows you to feel more comfortable with the unknown!

Adam J. Brown, M.D.

# Contents

*What is a Rheumatologist?* ..........................................................................................v

*Overview of this Book* ..............................................................................................vi

### Part I. Diagnosis and Treatment in Rheumatology

**Chapter 1     Evaluating the Patient with Joint Pain** .........................................................2

Inflammatory or Non-inflammatory? .......................................................................2

  *Inflammatory Arthritis* .............................................................................................2

    *Autoimmune Inflammatory Arthritis* ....................................................................2

    *Crystalline Arthritis* ..............................................................................................3

    *Infectious Arthritis* ...............................................................................................3

  *Non-inflammatory Arthritis* ...................................................................................3

    *Musculoskeletal Arthritis* .....................................................................................3

    *Osteoarthritis* ......................................................................................................3

    *Fibromyalgia. Central Pain* .................................................................................3

Location of the Joint Pain .......................................................................................3

How Many Joints Are Involved? .............................................................................4

  *Monoarticular Arthritis* ..........................................................................................4

  *Oligoarticular Arthritis* ..........................................................................................6

  *Polyarticular Arthritis* ............................................................................................6

Timeline and Pattern...............................................................................................6

Physical Examination of Inflammatory Joint Pain .................................................................. 6

Imaging and Laboratory in Joint Pain Evaluation ................................................................. 7

    *X-rays* ..................................................................................................................................... 7

    *Ultrasound* ............................................................................................................................. 7

    *MRI* ........................................................................................................................................ 7

    *Joint Fluid Examination* ....................................................................................................... 8

    *Blood Tests* ............................................................................................................................ 8

## Chapter 2    *The Immune System and Treatment in Rheumatology* .................... 9

Definitions ................................................................................................................................. 9

The Innate and Adaptive Immune Systems .......................................................................... 9

Non-Specific Anti-Rheumatic Medications ......................................................................... 10

    *NSAIDs* ................................................................................................................................ 11

    *Glucocorticoids* ................................................................................................................... 12

    *Disease-Modifying Anti-Rheumatic Drugs (DMARDs)* .................................................. 12

        *Anti-Malarial Drugs* ...................................................................................................... 12

        *Methotrexate* ................................................................................................................... 13

        *Azothioprine* ................................................................................................................... 13

        *Sulfasalazine* ................................................................................................................... 13

        *Leflunomide* .................................................................................................................... 14

        *Mycophenolate Mofetil* .................................................................................................. 14

        *Cyclophosphamide* .......................................................................................................... 14

Targeted Therapy ................................................................................................................... 14

    *TNF* ...................................................................................................................................... 14

    *Interleukin (IL) Inhibitors* ................................................................................................. 14

    *T-cell Interference* ............................................................................................................... 15

    *JAK/STAT Inhibitors* .......................................................................................................... 16

    *B-cell Depleting Therapies* ................................................................................................. 16

Other Immunosuppressive Drugs ........................................................................................ 16

    *Intravenous Immunoglobulin (IVIG)* ................................................................................ 16

    *Apremilast* ........................................................................................................................... 17

    *Dapsone* ............................................................................................................................... 17

    *Colchicine* ............................................................................................................................ 17

Overview of Immunosuppressive Medication in Autoimmune Diseases .......................... 17

# Part II. Inflammatory Arthritis

**Chapter 3  Rheumatoid Arthritis** ........................................................................ **20**

History in Rheumatoid Arthritis ........................................................................... 20

Physical Exam in Rheumatoid Arthritis ............................................................... 21

Extra-articular Manifestations of RA ................................................................... 22

    *Constitutional* ................................................................................................ 22

    *Rheumatoid Nodules* ..................................................................................... 22

    *Lung Disease* .................................................................................................. 22

    *Neck Instability* .............................................................................................. 22

    *Felty's Syndrome* ............................................................................................ 22

Laboratory Findings in Rheumatoid Arthritis .................................................... 22

Imaging Findings in Rheumatoid Arthritis ......................................................... 22

Treatment of Rheumatoid Arthritis ..................................................................... 23

Other Rheumatoid Arthritis-like Entities ........................................................... 24

    *Palindromic Rheumatoid Arthritis* ................................................................ 24

    *RS3PE* ........................................................................................................... 24

CASES ................................................................................................................... 24

**Chapter 4  Spondyloarthritis (SpA)** ................................................................. **25**

Ankylosing Spondylitis ........................................................................................ 25

Inflammatory Bowel Disease-Associated Arthritis ............................................ 26

Psoriatic Arthritis ................................................................................................. 26

Reactive Arthritis .................................................................................................. 26

    *Diagnosis of Reactive Arthritis* ..................................................................... 26

    *Treatment of Reactive Arthritis* ..................................................................... 27

History in Spondyloarthritis (SpA) ...................................................................... 27

    *Axial involvement in SpA* .............................................................................. 27

    *Peripheral involvement in SpA* ...................................................................... 27

Extra-articular Manifestations of SpA ................................................................ 28

Physical Exam in Spondyloarthritis .................................................................... 28

Laboratory and Imaging in Spondyloarthritis .................................................... 30

Treatment of SpA .................................................................................................. 30

CASES ................................................................................................................... 32

**Chapter 5     Systemic Lupus Erythematosus (SLE)** ...................................................**33**

History and Physical Exam in SLE ........................................................................ 33

Laboratory Diagnosis of SLE ............................................................................... 36

*Following a Patient with SLE* ....................................................................... 37

Differential Diagnosis of SLE .............................................................................. 37

*Drug-induced Lupus* .................................................................................... 37

*Antiphospholipid Syndrome* ........................................................................ 37

*Lupus Overlap Syndromes* ........................................................................... 38

Treatment of SLE ............................................................................................... 38

CASES ................................................................................................................ 38

**Chapter 6     Crystal Arthritis** ...........................................................................**40**

Gout .................................................................................................................. 40

*History in Gout* ........................................................................................... 41

*Laboratory in Gout* ..................................................................................... 41

*Serum Uric Acid* ................................................................................... 41

*Polarized microscopy* ............................................................................ 41

*X-ray* ................................................................................................... 42

*Treatment of Gout* ...................................................................................... 42

Pseudogout (CPPD) ........................................................................................... 43

*Pathophysiology of Pseudogout* ................................................................... 43

*History in Pseudogout* ................................................................................. 43

*Laboratory in Pseudogout* ........................................................................... 44

*Variations of Pseudogout* ............................................................................ 44

*Treatment of Pseudogout (CPPD)* ................................................................ 45

CASES ................................................................................................................ 45

**Chapter 7     Infectious Causes of Inflammatory Joint Pain** ..............................**47**

Septic Joint ........................................................................................................ 47

Infective Endocarditis ........................................................................................ 48

Migratory Inflammatory Arthritis ....................................................................... 48

Gonorrhea .......................................................................................................... 48

*Diagnosis and Treatment of Disseminated Gonococcus* ................................. 49

Rheumatic Fever ................................................................................................. 49

*Diagnosis of Rheumatic Fever* ..................................................................... 49

Organisms Causing Slowly Progressive Joint Damage ......................................... 50

*Mycobacterium Tuberculosis* ....................................................................... 50

     *Nontuberculous Mycobacterium*.................................................................................................50

     *Lyme Disease*.................................................................................................................................51

         *Diagnosis and Treatment of Lyme Disease*.......................................................................52

     *Whipple's Disease*.........................................................................................................................52

   Viral Causes of Inflammatory Arthritis...............................................................................................52

     *Parvovirus B19*.............................................................................................................................52

     *HIV*...............................................................................................................................................53

     *Hepatitis B*...................................................................................................................................53

     *Hepatitis C*...................................................................................................................................53

     *Chikungunya*................................................................................................................................53

     *Ross River Virus*..........................................................................................................................54

**Chapter 8     Autoinflammatory Disease**...........................................................................**56**

   Adult Onset Still's Disease (AOSD).....................................................................................................57

   Familial Mediterranean Fever..............................................................................................................58

   Tumor Necrosis Factor Receptor-1 Associated Periodic Syndrome (TRAPS)....................................58

   Hyperimmunoglobulin D Syndrome..................................................................................................59

   Cryopyrin-Associated Periodic Syndromes (CAPS)............................................................................59

     *Familial Cold Autoinflammatory Syndrome (FCAS)*......................................................................59

     *Muckle-Wells Syndrome (MWS)*....................................................................................................59

     *Neonatal-onset Multisystem Inflammatory Disease (NOMID)*.......................................................59

     *Treatment of CAPS*.....................................................................................................................60

   CASES.................................................................................................................................................60

**Part III. Non-Inflammatory Arthritis**

**Chapter 9     Osteoarthritis**...........................................................................................**63**

   History and Physical Exam in Osteoarthritis.......................................................................................63

   Laboratory and Imaging in Osteoarthritis...........................................................................................65

   Differential Diagnosis of Osteoarthritis...............................................................................................65

   Treatment of Osteoarthritis..................................................................................................................65

   CASES.................................................................................................................................................66

**Chapter 10   Fibromyalgia**............................................................................................**67**

   History in Fibromyalgia.......................................................................................................................67

   Physical Exam in Fibromyalgia...........................................................................................................67

   Treatment of Fibromyalgia..................................................................................................................68

   CASES.................................................................................................................................................68

# Part IV. Other Rheumatologic Diseases

*Chapter 11      Sjögren's Syndrome* ................................................................................**71**

History in Sjögren's Syndrome ................................................................................ 71

*Other Extra-Glandular Manifestations of Sjögren's* ................................................ 72

Physical Exam in Sjögren's Syndrome ........................................................................ 72

Laboratory in Sjögren's Syndrome ............................................................................ 73

Treatment of Sjögren's Syndrome ............................................................................ 73

CASE ........................................................................................................................ 73

*Chapter 12      Scleroderma* .................................................................................**75**

Pathophysiology of Scleroderma .............................................................................. 75

History in Scleroderma .............................................................................................. 75

Physical Exam in Scleroderma .................................................................................. 76

Categorizing Scleroderma ........................................................................................ 76

Laboratory Tests in Scleroderma .............................................................................. 77

Complications of Scleroderma .................................................................................. 78

Differential Diagnosis of Scleroderma ...................................................................... 78

Treatment of Scleroderma ........................................................................................ 79

CASES ...................................................................................................................... 79

*Chapter 13      Vasculitis* .....................................................................................**80**

Large Vessel Vasculitis .............................................................................................. 80

*Giant Cell Arteritis (Temporal Arteritis)* ................................................................ 80

*History in Giant Cell Arteritis* ................................................................................ 80

*Physical Exam in Giant Cell Arteritis* .................................................................... 81

*Diagnosis of GCA* .................................................................................................. 81

*Treatment of GCA* ................................................................................................ 81

*Polymyalgia Rheumatica* ...................................................................................... 81

*Takayasu's Arteritis* .............................................................................................. 82

Medium Vessel Vasculitis .......................................................................................... 83

*Polyarteritis Nodosa (PAN)* .................................................................................. 83

*History and Physical Exam in PAN* ........................................................................ 83

*Diagnosis of PAN* .................................................................................................. 83

*Treatment of PAN* ................................................................................................ 84

*Central Nervous System (CNS) Vasculitis* ............................................................ 84

*Reversible Cerebral Vasoconstriction Syndrome (RCVS)* ...................................... 84

*Behcet's Disease* .................................................................................................. 84

History and Physical Exam ................................................................................................ 84

Diagnosis of Behcet's Disease ........................................................................................... 85

Treatment of Behcet's Disease ........................................................................................... 85

ANCA-Associated Vasculitis (Small Blood Vessels) .............................................................. 85

Granulomatosis with Polyangiitis (GPA;Wegener's Disease) .............................................. 85

Microscopic Polyangiitis (MPA) ....................................................................................... 87

Goodpasture's Disease ...................................................................................................... 87

Eosinophilic Granulomatosis with Polyangiitis (EGPA; Churg-Strauss) ............................. 87

ANCA Not Associated with Vasculitis .................................................................................. 88

Medication-induced ANCA ............................................................................................... 88

Drug-induced ANCA ........................................................................................................ 88

Infection-induced ANCA .................................................................................................. 89

Cryoglobulinemic Vasculitis ............................................................................................... 89

CASES .................................................................................................................................. 89

**Chapter 14    Inflammatory Myopathies** .......................................................................... **91**

History in Inflammatory Myopathy ..................................................................................... 91

Polymyositis, Dermatomyositis, and Necrotizing Myopathy ................................................. 91

Physical Exam .................................................................................................................... 92

Diagnosis of Inflammatory Myopathy ............................................................................... 92

Other Causes of Muscle Weakness ..................................................................................... 93

Treatment of Inflammatory Myositis .................................................................................. 95

Inclusion Body Myositis ....................................................................................................... 95

Overlap Syndromes That Have Inflammatory Myopathy ...................................................... 95

Mixed Connective Tissue Disease (MCTD) ........................................................................ 95

Antisynthetase Syndrome .................................................................................................. 95

CASES .................................................................................................................................. 95

**Chapter 15    Miscellaneous Rheumatologic Diseases** ..................................................... **97**

Infiltrative Autoimmune Diseases ....................................................................................... 97

Sarcoidosis ......................................................................................................................... 97

IgG4-related Disease .......................................................................................................... 98

Granulomatosis with Polyangiitis ...................................................................................... 99

Rheumatoid Nodules .......................................................................................................... 99

Diffuse Lymphadenopathy .................................................................................................. 99

Castleman Disease ......................................................................................................... 99

Multicentric Castleman .............................................................................................. 99

Unicentric Castleman ................................................................................................. 100

*Autoimmune Lymphoproliferative Syndrome (ALPS)* ........................................................................ 100

*Diffuse Infiltrative Lymphocytosis Syndrome (DILS)* ..................................................................... 100

*Kukuchi Fujimoto Disease* ................................................................................................................ 100

*Autoimmune Eye Disease* .................................................................................................................. 100

    *Treatment of Autoimmune Eye Disease* ......................................................................................... 101

*Autoimmune Eye and Hearing Loss* ................................................................................................ 101

    *Cogan Syndrome* ............................................................................................................................ 101

    *Vogt-Koyanagi-Harada Disease* ................................................................................................... 101

    *Susac Disease* ................................................................................................................................ 101

*Relapsing Polychondritis* .................................................................................................................. 102

Osteoporosis and Osteopenia ............................................................................................................. 103

    *Diagnosis of Osteoporosis and Osteopenia* ................................................................................. 103

    *Treatment of Osteoporosis and Osteopenia* ................................................................................ 103

**Chapter 16   Pediatric Rheumatology** ............................................................................**104**

Bone/Joint Pain in a Pediatric Patient ............................................................................................... 104

    *Differential Diagnosis* ................................................................................................................... 104

Workup for Monoarticular Joint Pain in a Pediatric Patient ............................................................. 105

Autoimmune Arthritic Diseases in Pediatrics ................................................................................... 105

    *Systemic Juvenile Idiopathic Arthritis* .......................................................................................... 106

Autoimmune Juvenile Idiopathic Arthritis ....................................................................................... 106

    *Polyarticular Juvenile Idiopathic Arthritis* ................................................................................... 107

    *Oligoarticular Inflammatory Arthritis* .......................................................................................... 107

    *Enthesitis-related Juvenile Idiopathic Arthritis* ........................................................................... 108

    *Psoriatic Arthritis* ......................................................................................................................... 108

Medications in Pediatric Rheumatology ............................................................................................ 108

Common Non-inflammatory Causes of Pediatric Joint Pain ............................................................. 108

    *Chondromalacia patella* ............................................................................................................... 108

    *Osgood-Schlatter disease* ............................................................................................................. 108

    *Slipped capital femoral epiphysis* ................................................................................................ 108

    *Legg-Calve-Perthes disease* .......................................................................................................... 108

Pediatric Vasculitis ............................................................................................................................ 109

    *IgA Vasculitis (Henoch-Schönlein Purpura)* ................................................................................ 109

    *Kawasaki Disease* .......................................................................................................................... 110

CASES ................................................................................................................................................ 110

## Chapter 17 Antibodies and Other Lab Tests ................................................................. 111

Auto-antibodies ...............................................................................................................111

Anti-Nuclear Antibodies (ANA) .....................................................................................111

Anti-Double Stranded DNA Antibody (DS-DNA) & Anti-Smith Antibody ................. 112

All the Other Lupus Antibodies ...................................................................................... 112

    Anti-SSA/SSB (Ro/La) Antibody ............................................................................. 112

    Anti-Ribonucleoprotein (RNP) Antibody ................................................................ 112

    Anti-Histone Antibody ............................................................................................. 112

ANCA Antibodies ........................................................................................................... 113

Scleroderma Antibodies .................................................................................................. 113

    Anti-Centromere antibody ....................................................................................... 113

    Anti-SCL70/Topoisomerase antibody ...................................................................... 113

    RNA Polymerase III antibody ................................................................................. 113

Antisynthetase Antibodies ............................................................................................. 113

    Anti-JO-1 ................................................................................................................. 113

Rheumatoid Arthritis Antibodies ................................................................................... 114

    Rheumatoid Factor .................................................................................................. 114

    Anti CCP antibody .................................................................................................. 114

Other Rheumatologic Lab Tests ..................................................................................... 114

    ESR ........................................................................................................................... 114

    C-Reactive Protein .................................................................................................. 115

## Chapter 18 Rheumatology Review Questions ................................................................. 117

## INDEX .................................................................................................................................. 131

# Part I. Diagnosis and Treatment in Rheumatology

**1**

# Evaluating the Patient With Joint Pain

Joint pain is an extremely common complaint regardless of your field (as long as it's one where you're interacting with patients), so it is important to have a system that helps you sort through the differential diagnosis. At one end of the spectrum you have the 85-year-old man who worked in construction most of his life and presents with a 2-year history of right shoulder pain. At the other end is a 22-year-old African-American woman with a month-long history of morning stiffness in her ankles and wrists as well as swelling and tenderness in those joints. As you can imagine, both patients likely have very different causes for their joint pain and require different treatments. The history, physical exam, and laboratory tests play important roles in determining the diagnosis and treatment.

It's important to rule out trauma to a joint before working up a patient for autoimmune, crystalline, or infectious causes of joint pain. A badly twisted ankle or a broken big toe can look a lot like gout. The following descriptions of joint pain assume that no trauma occurred to the joint.

## Inflammatory or Non-Inflammatory?

When joint pain occurs with no precipitating event (obvious injury to the joint), it can be divided into *inflammatory* or *non-inflammatory joint pain*. *Inflammatory joint pain* occurs when the immune system causes an inflammatory infiltrate made up of multiple types of immune cells (macrophages, neutrophils, monocytes) in the joint tissue, resulting in swelling and pain in the affected joint. Multiple etiologies can trigger joint inflammation, namely autoimmune diseases, crystalline disease (gout), or infection. In contrast, *non-inflammatory joint pain* is not caused by the immune system infiltrating a joint, e.g. musculoskeletal arthritis (rotator cuff injury, tendon tear, and ligament injury), osteoarthritis, or fibromyalgia. Non-inflammatory joint pain is much more common than inflammatory joint pain.

## Inflammatory Arthritis

*Inflammatory arthritis* implies the immune system is acting within the joint to cause the swelling and pain the patient is experiencing. Inflammatory joint pain can arise from autoimmune diseases, crystalline disease, or infection. Remember, for the discussion of inflammatory arthritis, we assume the patient's joint pain occurs spontaneously, and not following any sort of trauma.

***Autoimmune inflammatory arthritis.*** The immune system attacks the joints, causing joint swelling and pain. There are multiple causes, classic examples being *rheumatoid arthritis*, *systemic lupus erythematosus*, and *spondyloarthritis*. Which joint is affected depends on the disease; generally, *patients describe joint pain and swelling that is worse in the mornings and gets better the more they use the joint(s).* This is a distinct description of autoimmune joint pain. Other kinds of joint pain, especially those of mechanical origin (like osteoarthritis), almost always get worse the more the patient uses the joint.

*Crystalline arthritis,* most commonly *gout,* is an extremely painful condition that doesn't present the same way as autoimmune inflammatory arthritis. The pain of crystalline arthritis usually develops rapidly and seemingly out of the blue in one or more joints. The patient may describe waking up with a swollen, extremely tender toe. This joint pain is usually much worse with activity, but it can be distinguished from non-inflammatory joint pain because the affected joint is usually very swollen, very warm and extremely tender to palpation; and the patient's range of motion is severely limited. Over the course of a few days, more joints may become involved. The immune system is reacting to crystals within the joint, which causes the severe swelling. In contrast, in an autoimmune disease, the immune system would be targeting its own synovial lining of the joint. (For more, see Chapter 6, Crystal Arthritis.)

*Infectious arthritis* can appear identical to crystalline arthritis but is almost always monoarticular. The joint is red, hot, and swollen. The patient won't be able to move the joint because of the pain. Evaluating joint fluid can help distinguish crystalline arthritis from infectious arthritis, since the white blood cell count in gout will usually be between 2,000 and 50,000 cells/mm$^3$, while the WBC count in infection will often exceed 50,000/mm$^3$.

## Non-inflammatory Arthritis

*Non-Inflammatory arthritis* is by far the more common cause of joint pain. Usually there is a minimal amount of swelling or warmth of the joint. In non-inflammatory arthritis, the pain is worse as the day progresses and the more the joints are used. The most common causes of non-inflammatory joint pain are:

*Musculoskeletal arthritis.* This group includes a broad range of injuries, including rotator cuff injury, tendon tear, and ligament injury. These types usually occur after direct injury or repetitive motion to a certain joint and are usually monoarticular; symptoms worsen with activity. Rarely, there can be a tear in the muscle/tendon, causing bleeding in the joint, which will produce visible joint swelling.

*Osteoarthritis (OA).* This is the "wear and tear" arthritis most of the population will develop with age. OA typically affects the distal interphalangeal, proximal interphalangeal, and carpal metacarpal joints **(Fig. 1-1)**, as well as the knees and hips. Patients often describe pain worsening the more they use the affected joint and may note mild swelling of the joint, especially the knees, but the swelling is not warm or tender to the touch (see Chapter 9, Osteoarthritis).

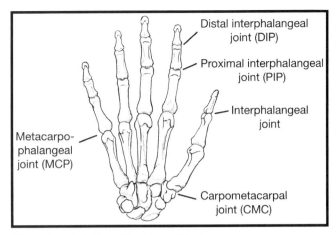

*Figure 1-1.* Labeling of the joints of the hand.

*Fibromyalgia. Central pain* is most commonly seen in fibromyalgia. This pain is usually described as "all over" body pain. Both muscles and joints are affected. The patients will often say they feel swollen, but their joints don't actually appear swollen. Almost always the pain gets worse with activity and is accompanied by severe fatigue. (See Chapter 10, Fibromyalgia.)

## Location of the Joint Pain

When evaluating a patient with joint pain, it's critical to note which joint or joints are involved. Certain diseases, for uncertain reasons, prefer particular joints. For example, if the patient wakes up with a swollen and extremely tender big toe, your first thought will be gout. This is an example of pattern recognition, which rheumatologists and other health care providers employ every day in the clinic to make a diagnosis; location of the joint pain is an important component of the overall pattern of disease presentation. Although rheumatologic diseases can present in a wide variety of locations, the following are examples of classic joint involvement and associated diseases.

### Hands

*Metacarpophalangeal joints (MCPs).* If the primary site of hand pain is the MCPs, an inflammatory cause should be higher on your differential, whether autoimmune (e.g. rheumatoid arthritis); crystalline such as gout/pseudogout; or infectious such as parvovirus. Primary osteoarthritis rarely involves the MCPs. If there is evidence of OA in the MCPs, think of secondary causes of OA such as hemochromatosis or pseudogout (see Chapter 9, Osteoarthritis). The takeaway is: If the MCPs are the primary location of joint pain, workup should be done evaluating for inflammatory causes of joint pain **(see Figs. 1-2, 1-3 for overview of location of hand pain)**.

*Proximal interphalangeal joints (PIPs).* These joints are in the gray area of diagnostic workup. The diseases

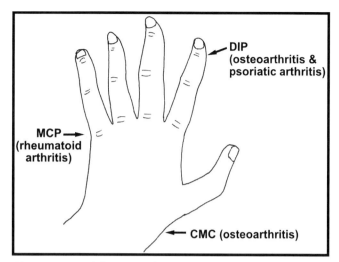

*Figure 1-2 Hand drawing indicating the joints that have a predilection for certain disease presentations. CMC=Carpal Metacarpal joint; DIP= Distal Interphalangeal joint; MCP=Metacarpal Phalangeal joint.*

that mostly affect the MCPs can also involve the PIPs, and the diseases that affect the DIPs can also involve the PIPs (OA of the PIPs presents as bony enlargement referred to as a *Bouchard node*). If the main symptom is PIP joint pain, location doesn't help as much, and you need to rely more on the history and physical exam to make a diagnosis.

*Distal Interphalangeal joints (DIPs).* DIP pain is most commonly non-inflammatory, but in rare instances autoimmune diseases can involve the DIP:

- Non-inflammatory DIP pain. Osteoarthritis (OA) is by far the most common cause of DIP pain. OA presents as bony enlargement *(Heberden's nodes)* and a dull ache of the DIPs that worsens with activity. Bony enlargement can be mistaken for swelling, but you'll note the joint is hard like a bone on exam, and the patient will say the swelling doesn't fluctuate—it's just always enlarged.
- Inflammatory DIP pain. The inflammatory arthritis that favors the DIPs is *spondyloarthritis,* particularly *psoriatic arthritis* (see Chapter 4, Spondyloarthritis). It's possible to differentiate

psoriatic arthritis from OA based on history and physical exam. Patients with psoriatic arthritis are usually younger, and the pain and swelling come and go as the day progresses, improving with activity; whereas OA has permanent bony enlargement and mostly persistent pain that worsens with activity.

*The Carpometacarpal (CMC).* The CMC joint is the joint at the base of the thumb and is predisposed to developing OA. Older patients often complain of pain at the base of their thumbs, often making it difficult to open jars. On physical exam, the CMC may bulge laterally, termed *"squaring of the CMC"* (see Chapter 9, Osteoarthritis).

### Feet

*Big toe.* Swelling and severe pain in the *big toe* is a classic description of gout *"podagra."* Gout can affect many different joints but tends to attack the big toe first.

*Metatarsal phalangeal joints (MTPs)* are often involved in rheumatoid arthritis. The 5th *toe ("pinky toe")* is usually the first joint to develop erosions on x-ray in rheumatoid arthritis.

## How Many Joints Are Involved?

Whether one or multiple joints are inflamed changes the diagnostic possibilities and how to proceed with the workup (**Fig. 1-4**).

*Monoarticular arthritis.* When a patient has one large swollen joint, rule out infection as quickly as possible. Crystalline disease is a more common cause of monoarticular joint pain than infection, but an infection can quickly cause irreversible joint destruction if not recognized and treated promptly.

The patient's age is important in diagnosing monoarticular joint pain. Older patients are much more likely to have crystalline disease than younger patients. Another factor that increases the likelihood of crystalline disease is the history of a previous similar attack, suggesting disease recurrence. The history may increase the likelihood that the joint pain represents gout, but unfortunately there isn't anything on history,

| FIGURE 1-3 HAND JOINTS IN RHEUMATIC CONDITIONS | | | | |
|---|---|---|---|---|
| | **MCP** | **PIP** | **DIP** | **CMC** |
| **Non-Inflammatory** | | Osteoarthritis (Bouchard Node) | Osteoarthritis (Heberden's Node) | Osteoarthritis (Squaring of the CMC) |
| **Autoimmune Inflammatory** | Rheumatoid Arthritis | Rheumatoid Arthritis/ Spondyloarthritis | Spondyloarthritis | |
| **Crystalline Disease** | Gout/Pseudogout | Gout/Pseudogout | Gout/Pseudogout | |

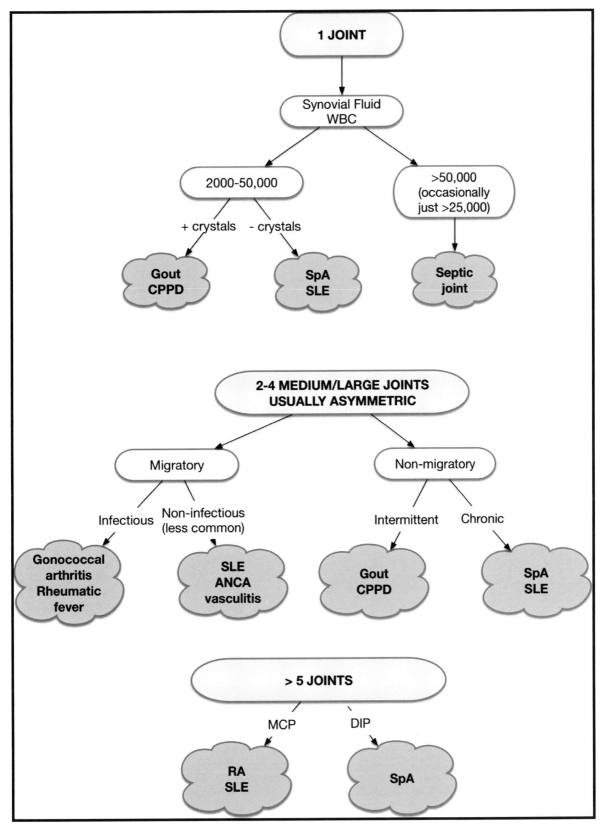

***Figure 1-4*** *Simplified flow chart of conditions to consider when evaluating a patient, based on the number of joints involved at presentation. ANCA vasculitis = Antineutrophil Cytoplasmic Antibody vasculitis; CPPD =Calcium Pyrophosphate Deposition; RA = Rheumatoid Arthritis; SLE = Systemic Lupus Erythematosus; SpA = Spondyloarthritis; WBC=White Blood Cell.*

physical exam, or blood tests that conclusively rules out infections. Tapping the joint (*arthrocentesis*) and examining the fluid are critical in distinguishing infections from other causes.

Another cause of monoarticular arthritis is early spondyloarthritis, which may begin in a medium joint like an elbow or a large joint such as the knee. The disease can start with monoarticular involvement, then over weeks to months add additional joints (see Chapter 4, Spondyloarthritis).

*Oligoarticular arthritis* refers to 2-4 joints involved. Oligoarticular arthritis usually refers to the medium (wrist, elbows, ankles) and large (shoulders, hips, knees) joints. It would be unusual for 2-4 fingers to be involved (if the fingers are involved it's usually polyarticular). Oligoarticular inflammatory arthritis is also often asymmetric; for example, a patient presents with a swollen, tender left wrist and right ankle.

Oligoarticular involvement is consistent with *spondyloarthritis*, as well as certain types of *vasculitis*. Infectious oligoarticular arthritis is seen *with Lyme disease* and *gonococcal arthritis*.

It is important to classify oligoarticular arthritis as *symmetric* or *asymmetric*. Why? If the patient has symmetric bilateral wrist swelling and pain, this may be early rheumatoid arthritis; and if enough time passes, the fingers will become involved, developing into a polyarticular arthritis. If the oligoarticular arthritis is asymmetric, it is less likely to become polyarticular.

*Polyarticular arthritis* usually means that 5 or more joints are involved. Again, location and symmetry are important in working up polyarticular disease. If the MCPs are involved, it's more likely rheumatoid arthritis. If the DIPs are involved, it's more likely psoriatic arthritis or osteoarthritis. Symmetric polyarticular inflammatory arthritis is consistent with rheumatoid arthritis, and asymmetric polyarticular inflammatory arthritis could be spondyloarthritis.

## Timeline and Pattern

The timeline of the joint pain commonly guides you in diagnosis. How long has the pain been ongoing? Did the patient do anything to cause the pain? In what pattern did the joint pain progress: migratory, additive, or intermittent?

*How long has the pain been ongoing?* If a symmetric polyarticular inflammatory arthritis that looks just like rheumatoid arthritis presents with only 3 weeks of pain, this could be a viral illness or a post-viral reactive arthritis that is self-limited and doesn't require prolonged immunosuppression. Unless there is strong evidence of an underlying autoimmune disease (positive anti-CCP antibody), it's usually a good idea to wait 6 weeks to see if the symptoms resolve before initiating long-term immunosuppression.

*Repetitive movements* over a long period of time can produce micro tears in the tendons, causing mild inflammation and pain. For example, someone who paints houses for a living and positions his arm above his head all day may present with shoulder pain. The pain in this situation usually comes on slowly and worsens over time. The patient will usually inform the physician if trauma was involved. Thus, a patient presenting with a swollen ankle may tell you he "twisted" it while playing basketball.

There may be *no history of precipitating events*. This is the joint pain that just starts "out of nowhere." It may start slowly with occasional pain, but over months to years the pain becomes more persistent, as in knee osteoarthritis. Or it can be 10/10 pain that starts immediately when the patient wakes up in the morning, as we see in gout and other crystalline diseases.

The *pattern of joint involvement* refers to how the joints became involved. Did the pain start in one joint, then more and more joints became involved (additive)? Or did the joint pain start in one joint, spontaneously resolve, then move to another joint (migratory)?

An *additive pattern* happens when a patient starts experiencing joint pain in one or two joints, later involving additional joints. This is the most common pattern in a number of autoimmune diseases, such as rheumatoid arthritis. Pain may start in a patient's metacarpal phalangeal joints. A few weeks later the wrist and elbows become involved. Eventually the patient will see the physician with multiple joints flaring all at once.

A *migratory pattern* is when the patient experiences pain in one joint, which eventually resolves, only to have a different joint become involved. The patient may present with one or two joints flaring, but will say that earlier a few other joints were involved that now look normal. Classic examples of this are *rheumatic fever* and *gonococcal arthritis*, but it can also occur in other diseases, such as *systemic lupus erythematosus, sarcoidosis, early Lyme disease*, and certain types of *vasculitis*.

*Intermittent arthritis* refers to one or more joints becoming swollen and painful, then spontaneously resolving, then recurring weeks to months later. This is a classic pattern in crystalline diseases such as gout.

## Physical Examination of Inflammatory Joint Pain

*Synovitis* means inflammation around the joint's synovial lining (**Fig. 1-5**). It takes some practice to appreciate synovitis on exam, especially in a small joint like the MCP. The joint appears puffy ("boggy" on

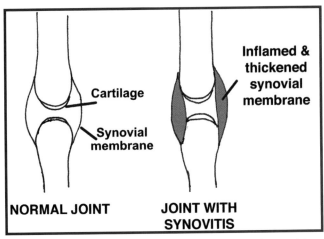

*Figure 1-5* *Anatomy of a normal joint and a joint with synovitis. Notice the synovial thickening.*

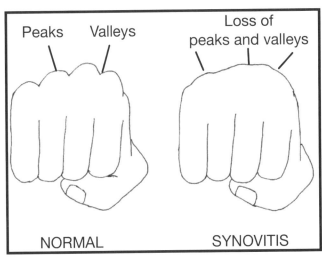

*Figure 1-6* *Physical exam of a normal hand making a fist and that of a patient who has synovitis in the metacarpal phalangeal joints.*

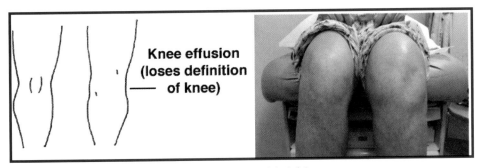

*Figure 1- 7* *Knee effusion. Notice the loss of definition of the left knee.*

palpation, with a warm spongy feel), not as well defined as its contralateral brethren when compared on physical exam. If the MCPs are involved, the joints will lose definition of the knuckles when the patient makes a fist, and the examiner won't be able to appreciate the peaks and valleys of the knuckles **(Fig. 1-6)**.

*Effusion* is when a joint has excess fluid within it. The best way to tell this is to visually compare the affected joint with the same joint on the opposite side and then palpate the joint. You should be able to see a difference in the size and the overall look of the joint when compared side-by-side. When you palpate the joint, you can sometimes feel the fluid being pushed from one side of the joint to the other. The knee is the best example of this **(Fig. 1-7)**.

# Imaging and Laboratory in Joint Pain Evaluation

*X-rays* are usually the first imaging step in evaluating a patient with joint pain. X-rays are limited as they don't visualize soft tissue well, but they will reveal major bony changes that can give diagnostic clues, such as a fracture. If a patient has a severe inflammatory arthritis, bony erosions can be seen where chunks of the bone around the joint have been eaten away, but this usually takes months to years to develop. This differs from osteoarthritis, where an x-ray shows bony enlargement (*osteophytes*) and asymmetric joint space narrowing without erosions.

*Ultrasound* is an imaging modality that can be used at the bedside by a practitioner skilled in its use. It is noninvasive and relatively inexpensive compared to MRI. Ultrasound can detect joint effusions, tenosynovitis, and—depending on the skill of the examiner—tendon tears. When ultrasound is used on the hands, erosions of the bones can also be detected, giving a clue to the diagnosis. Ultrasound training is becoming more common in rheumatology fellowship training.

*MRI* is a much more expensive imaging modality, but you can get better images of synovitis, tendon inflammation, effusions, and masses with an MRI than with x-rays or ultrasound.

*Joint fluid examination*, draining fluid from the joint (*arthrocentesis*) and examining it, is critical in the workup and diagnosis of patients with underlying autoimmune disease. The physician can quickly distinguish inflammatory vs non-inflammatory, and infectious vs non-infectious fluid on synovial fluid exam. If the synovial fluid is clear and you can read a newspaper behind it, the fluid is unlikely to be inflammatory and much less likely to be infected. If the fluid is murky and difficult to see through, it's likely inflammatory and possibly infectious. The lab should analyze the fluid and report the approximate number of white blood cells in the fluid (this can also be done by the physician with a microscope). The classic number you should worry about is a white blood cell count of greater than $50,000/mm^3$, which greatly increases the likelihood of an infectious etiology. It is important to note, though, that septic arthritis can also be seen with white blood cell counts as low as $25,000/mm^3$, but if it's higher than $50,000/mm^3$, infection should be much higher on the differential. If the white blood cell count is somewhere between 2,000 and $50,000/mm^3$, then gout or an autoimmune cause is possible. If the WBC is less than $2,000/mm^3$, a non-inflammatory cause like osteoarthritis is more likely **(Fig. 1-8)**.

*Blood tests* are also very important, depending on the disease(s) under consideration and will be discussed in relation to specific diseases.

| FIGURE 1-8 SYNOVIAL FLUID ANALYSIS | | | |
|---|---|---|---|
| **Type of Joint Disease** | **Osteoarthritis** | **Autoimmune inflammatory arthritis and crystalline disease** | **Septic Joint** |
| **White Blood Cell Count** | $<2,000/mm^3$ | $2,000-50,000/mm^3$ | $>50,000/mm^3$ (but can be seen in $>25,000/mm^3$) |

# 2

# The Immune System and Treatment in Rheumatology

The field of rheumatology and the treatments it employs deal in large part with dysfunction of the immune system. This chapter provides a brief overview of the functions of the immune system and the effects of immunosuppressive medications used in a variety of diseases discussed throughout the book.

The immune system is complex and far from being fully elucidated. Every year more knowledge accumulates about the numerous cells involved as well as the complex interactions between the cells and their products. The more knowledge gained about the immune system, the better we can understand the pathophysiology of autoimmune diseases, which can provide potential targets for newer drug therapies. This is one of the most exciting aspects of rheumatology; every year more medications are approved for the treatment of an array of autoimmune diseases.

## Definitions

*Cytokine* is a generic term used to describe any substance secreted by immune cells that allows an interaction to occur between cells. Examples of cytokines are *interferons*, *interleukins*, and *tumor necrosis factor (TNF)*.

*Interleukin.* There are many types of interleukins that are secreted by many types of cells of the immune system. Interleukins are glycoproteins that were first discovered to be secreted by leukocytes (white blood cells), hence the term *interleukin.* However, it is now known that interleukins are secreted by a variety of cell types. A few select interleukins are thought to play a prominent role in the pathophysiology of multiple autoimmune diseases.

*Tumor necrosis factor (TNF)* is involved in multiple pathways, including fevers, inflammation, and cell death. TNF was originally named because of its ability to kill certain cancer cells. It was later discovered to be involved in a multitude of immune processes and is secreted by a variety of immune cells.

## The Innate and Adaptive Immune Systems

We can simplify the immune system by dividing it into the *innate immune system* and the *adaptive immune system* **(Fig. 2-1).** In reality, these are not truly segregated systems; one cannot function appropriately without the other, and the two systems enhance one another. Both systems are complex, and few of the rheumatologic medications or diseases can be classified as only involving one aspect of the immune system versus the other.

*The innate immune system* is the first line of defense again infectious organisms. The innate immune system acts quickly; cells recognize foreign invaders, kill the invaders, and then signal other cells to respond

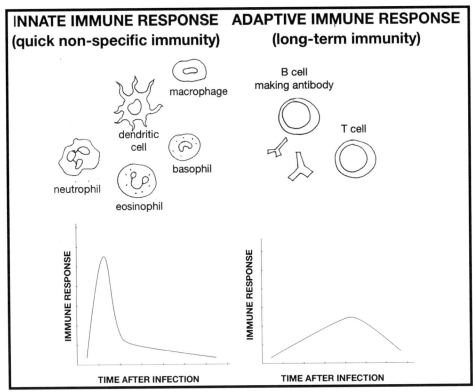

**INNATE IMMUNE RESPONSE**
(quick non-specific immunity)

**ADAPTIVE IMMUNE RESPONSE**
(long-term immunity)

macrophage

dendritic cell

neutrophil

basophil

eosinophil

B cell making antibody

T cell

IMMUNE RESPONSE

TIME AFTER INFECTION

IMMUNE RESPONSE

TIME AFTER INFECTION

*Figure 2-1* *Cells involved in the innate and adaptive immune system and their activity levels in relation to the time of infection.*

and kill more of the infectious organisms. The innate immune system is comprised of a variety of cell types, including cells that phagocytize other cells (neutrophils, macrophages, and dendritic cells) and cells that specialize in cell signaling. The innate immune system reacts quickly to eliminate an infectious threat by coordinating signals from cells that recognize the infectious organism to cells that phagocytose and eliminate the threat.

*The adaptive immune system* steps in if the innate immune system fails to extinguish the infectious threat. The adaptive system remembers previous infections through the production of antibodies. Vaccines work by stimulating the adaptive immune system to provide long-term immune memory. The adaptive immune system is highly complex and not fully elucidated. For simplicity, we will focus on two major cells of the adaptive immune system, B and T cells, which are manipulated by immunosuppressive medications.

*B Cells.* The B cell is a lymphocyte that matures in the bone marrow (hence, B for bone marrow). B cells produce *antibodies*, which are pivotal for immunologic memory. Antibodies are protein complexes formed after the immune system has been exposed to a particular infectious organism (bacteria or virus). Once the B cell has been exposed to the organism, the B cell matures into a *plasma cell,* which produces large quantities of antibodies for years. Later, when the antibodies react to

the same infectious organism, an inflammatory response will occur immediately.

*T Cells.* T cells are lymphocytes that mature in the thymus (hence, T for thymus). Multiple types of T cells exist, each performing specific duties. The primary types of T cells are *cytotoxic T cells* and *helper T cells.* Cytotoxic T cells destroy cells infected with viruses, as well as cancer cells and damaged cells. T helper cells are divided into *T helper cell 1 (Th1)* and *T helper cell 2 (Th2)* types. These cells assist other cells and are involved in cell signaling. All T cells start from naive T cells which, depending on the cytokines they are exposed to, differentiate into mature T cells that have specific functions. It is important to know how the different subsets of T cells are formed because specific medications block certain cytokines that are needed for T cell subsets to develop **(Fig. 2-2)**.

# Nonspecific Anti-Rheumatic Medications

The following are immunosuppressive drugs with nonspecific mechanisms of action. This contrasts with newer agents that block a specific cytokine in the inflammatory pathway. The older immunosuppressives likely suppress both the innate and adaptive immune

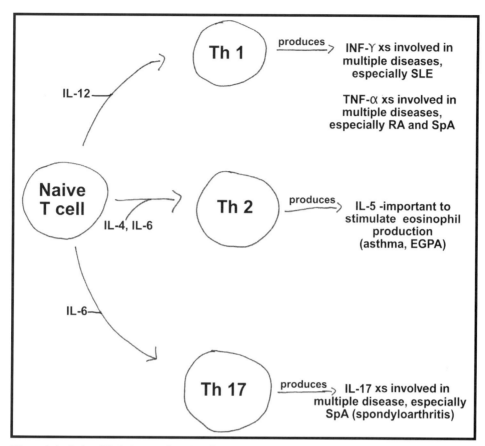

*Figure 2-2  A simplified picture of T cell differentiation. (xs = excess)*

systems, but the mechanism of how these anti-rheumatic medications treat autoimmune diseases isn't completely clear.

*Non-steroidal anti-Inflammatory drugs (NSAIDs)* and *Glucocorticoids (steroids)* are considered backbone therapy for a number of autoimmune diseases. They are rarely used by themselves, but are used in combination with other longer-acting medications.

## *Non-steroidal Anti-inflammatory Drugs (NSAIDs)*

*Non-steroidal anti-inflammatory drugs (NSAIDs)* are used to rapidly decrease inflammation **(Fig. 2-3)**. These drugs are widely used for a variety of conditions, even non-inflammatory conditions, such as osteoarthritis (see Chapter 9, Osteoarthritis). NSAIDs exert their effect by inhibiting cyclooxygenases (COX-1 and COX-2), both of which are important in the inflammatory cascade. NSAIDs are not given as long-term monotherapy in autoimmune disease, since they are not thought to be potent enough to actually halt the disease progression or stop damage to the joints. NSAIDs are often given as an adjuvant to other treatments, to minimize pain from the underlying disease.

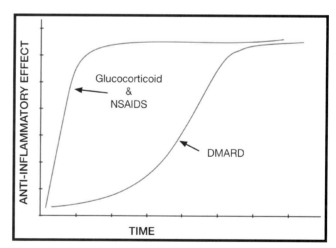

*Figure 2-3  Note the rapid anti-inflammatory effect of NSAIDs and glucocorticoids in contrast to DMARDs, which have a much slower onset of action.*

To understand the toxicities of NSAIDs, it is important to note what COX-1 and COX-2 do:

- **COX-1** is found in virtually all cells. It is important for the production of prostaglandins, which protect the gastric lining of the stomach (NSAIDs increase risk of gastric ulcers), affect platelet aggregation

(NSAIDs increase risk of bleeding), and regulate vasodilation of the blood vessels to the kidneys (NSAIDs can cause kidney damage, especially in patients with poor renal function; NSAIDs should be avoided in patients with chronic kidney disease).

- *COX-2* is more specifically found in the inflamed synovium of rheumatoid arthritis patients, and less in other tissues. This fact suggests that if COX-2 were more specifically targeted, the drug would have fewer side effects than the combined COX-1/COX-2 inhibitor. This, however, has not proven true. COX-2 inhibitors have also been shown to be associated with gastric ulcers and kidney injury.

## Glucocorticoids

*Glucocorticoids*, like NSAIDs, exert their anti-inflammatory effect rapidly, relieving inflammation within hours of taking the drugs. Glucocorticoids are the backbone of treatment in most autoimmune diseases. If a patient presents with a new diagnosis of rheumatoid arthritis, with swollen painful joints, none of the drugs mentioned below will give the patient relief within the next few days. Glucocorticoids, however, will decrease the swelling and pain within hours. Glucocorticoids can be given at high doses (prednisone 40-60 mg/day), moderate doses (prednisone 20-40 mg/day), or low doses (prednisone less than 20 mg/day), depending on the severity of the disease. Glucocorticoids are given in conjunction with a longer-term "steroid-sparing" anti-rheumatic drug, which may take months to start exerting its effect and decreasing inflammation. Glucocorticoids are usually started at a higher dose and then tapered over the course of weeks to months.

Importantly, if the patient is on prednisone more than 10 mg a day for more than 10 days, the dose should not be stopped abruptly, but slowly tapered to zero, because the body normally makes its own prednisone equivalent of about 5-7 mg a day. When the body is exposed to exogenous glucocorticoid for a period of more than 10 days, it will decrease endogenous production of the steroid. So if the prednisone is stopped abruptly, the body will not make its own steroid, which is important for maintaining glucose levels and blood pressure. As a result of the abrupt halt of steroids, the patient's blood pressure may decrease to life-threatening levels.

Glucocorticoids cannot be used long-term, at least not at moderate to high doses. Their side effects are numerous and inevitable with prolonged use. The more common side effects include weight gain and redistribution of weight. Patients will display a *Cushingoid* appearance, including *moon facies*, which is fat distribution in the cheeks, with swelling of the face. Fat can also accumulate in the upper back of patients, giving a hunchback appearance. The skin of patients on long-term glucocorticoids will also thin, causing easy bruising as well as purplish stretch marks on the abdomen. Other side effects include elevated blood sugar (which can become dangerously elevated, especially in patients with diabetes), elevated blood pressure, as well as weakening of the bones (*osteopenia* and *osteoporosis*). If patients are on prolonged glucocorticoid treatment, they should undergo a bone mineral density scan to measure the strength of their bones.

## Disease-Modifying Anti-Rheumatic Drugs (DMARDs)

*Disease-Modifying Anti-Rheumatic Drugs (DMARDs)* are a category of unrelated medications used for a variety of autoimmune conditions. These medications have been around for decades, and many of them were originally used to treat different types of cancer. It wasn't until much later in the history of the drugs that they were used to treat autoimmune diseases.

Unlike NSAIDS and steroids, which treat the acute inflammation but do not prevent progression of disease, DMARDs may slow down the progression of the disease through a variety of mechanisms that inhibit the production of more cells (cellular turnover). We think the decrease in cell turnover inhibits the production of inflammatory cells that would produce more damage to the joints, but just how DMARDs prevent damage in autoimmune diseases isn't totally understood.

The side-effect profiles of DMARDs are similar. The bone marrow produces different kinds of cells, including white blood cells and red blood cells. When DMARDs are taken, the bone marrow may have more difficulty producing these cells, so patients on these medications need to have monthly blood tests to evaluate for low white blood cells, low hemoglobin, or low platelets. If a low level is detected, the dose of the drug can be decreased, or the drug may be stopped, depending on the severity of the low count. If the patient does not have labs checked for a long period of time, the white blood count may decrease to dangerously low levels, making the patient susceptible to infection. See **Figure 2-4** for a summary of DMARD therapies.

It's important to note that DMARD therapy often takes months to start working, so a patient should not expect a rapid resolution of symptoms when initiating these medications. NSAIDs and glucocorticoids, which relieve symptoms rapidly, can be used at the same time as initiating DMARD therapy to provide relief while the DMARD starts to take effect **(Fig. 2-3).**

### Anti-malarial Drugs

You may wonder why medications used to treat malaria have been adopted by rheumatologists to treat

| FIGURE 2-4 TRADITIONAL DISEASE-MODIFYING ANTI-RHEUMATIC DRUGS | | | | |
|---|---|---|---|---|
| | Mechanism of Action | Administration | Safety Surveillance | Contraindications |
| **Hydroxychloroquine (Plaquenil)** | Anti-malarial | Oral once to twice daily | Ophthalmologic exam yearly | Retinal disease |
| **Methotrexate** | Anti-metabolite, decreases DNA synthesis | Oral given weekly, or subcutaneous | CBC and CMP monthly | Renal or liver impairment |
| **Azathioprine (Imuran)** | Decreases DNA synthesis | Oral given daily | CBC and CMP monthly | Renal impairment |
| **Sulfasalazine** | Decreases prostaglandin synthesis | Oral given twice a day | CBC and CMP monthly | Sulfa-allergic |
| **Leflunomide** | Inhibits DNA synthesis | Oral given daily | CBC and CMP monthly | Severe hepatic impairment |
| **Mycophenolate mofetil (Cellcept)** | Inhibits B and T cell proliferation | Oral given twice daily | CBC and CMP monthly | |
| CBC = Complete Blood Count; CMP = Complete Metabolic Profile | | | | |

autoimmune diseases. The story originates in World War II, when soldiers stationed in the Pacific were given anti-malarial medications to prevent malaria. Soldiers with rheumatoid arthritis and systemic lupus erythematous started to feel better, and it was hypothesized that the improvement was because of the prophylactic anti-malarials. Subsequent studies showed modest efficacy for systemic lupus erythematosus with very minimal risk of side effects. The most commonly prescribed anti-malarial for autoimmune disease treatment is *hydroxychloroquine (Plaquenil)*. Anti-malarials have become a backbone treatment in many autoimmune diseases, especially systemic lupus erythematosus, because they offer mild benefit with minimal side effects. Anti-malarials are by far the safest drugs rheumatologists prescribe, so there is often a low threshold to prescribe them.

The most concerning side effect is pigment deposition in the retina. This deposition will be found by ophthalmologists prior to any vision loss as long as the patient is being seen regularly. Also, the deposition usually takes more than 5 years of constant use of the drug to actually cause problems. As long as the patient on the anti-malarial drug is seen once a year by an ophthalmologist, the drug would be very unlikely to have a significant adverse reaction.

*Methotrexate* is first-line treatment for patients with rheumatoid arthritis, as well as many diseases, such as systemic lupus erythematosus and multiple forms of vasculitis. Methotrexate was originally used for leukemia, as it blocks the synthesis of rapidly dividing cells that are seen in cancer. It wasn't until decades later that methotrexate was used to treat rheumatoid arthritis and shown to be effective, likely due to a complex anti-inflammatory effect. Methotrexate also depletes the body of folic acid, so folic acid is often given along with the medication.

Because of the use of methotrexate in cancer, patients who are prescribed methotrexate for rheumatoid arthritis may investigate the drug on the internet and wonder why they are receiving chemotherapy for an autoimmune disease. It is important to stress to these patients that the dosage of methotrexate for cancer therapy is significantly higher than the dose given by rheumatologists; the dose given by rheumatologists has significantly fewer side effects.

Methotrexate should be avoided in patients with liver or kidney disease.

*Azathioprine (Imuran),* like methotrexate, decreases the amount of DNA synthesis in cells, thus inhibiting the production of new cells (cell turnover). As with methotrexate, it was originally used to treat malignancy. It was later discovered to decrease the amount of antibodies produced in response to certain infectious organisms. Because of this discovery, azathioprine was first used in transplant medicine to decrease the transplant recipient's immune system's ability to reject the transplanted organ. The drug is now used in a variety of diseases, such as systemic lupus erythematosus and as maintenance therapy (but not induction therapy, which is the more aggressive treatment given at initial diagnosis) for different types of vasculitis.

*Sulfasalazine* is the first drug to be synthesized specifically to treat rheumatoid arthritis. (The other DMARDs were made for another indication and later discovered to also work for rheumatoid arthritis.) It was originally designed in 1938 with the idea that infection was the cause of rheumatoid arthritis; thus, the antibacterial sulfa aspect of the drug. Rheumatoid arthritis was later shown to be an autoimmune disease, but the drug had clinical efficacy despite not being used for the original intention. Sulfasalazine undergoes multiple conversions once it's absorbed, and it's unclear which aspect of the drug is actually an anti-inflammatory agent and works for autoimmune diseases.

*Leflunomide,* as with methotrexate and azathioprine, exerts its effects by inhibiting DNA synthesis, but why exactly this helps with autoimmune diseases is not clear. Leflunomide can be used in patients with kidney disease.

*Mycophenolate mofetil (Cellcept)* is a more recent DMARD. Unlike the other DMARDs, this drug isn't used in rheumatoid arthritis. Its first use was to reduce rejection in patients with renal transplants. Mycophenolate mofetil's primary use in autoimmune disease is treating renal involvement in systemic lupus erythematosus. It has also been used in patients with interstitial lung disease secondary to systemic autoimmune diseases like scleroderma.

### Alkylating Agent

*Cyclophosphamide,* like other immunosuppressant drugs, was originally manufactured as a chemotherapeutic agent to treat malignancy by stopping cell division in rapidly dividing cells. Its mechanism in autoimmune disease is not completely understood. Cyclophosphamide, arguably the most potent of the immunosuppressive medications, is used in a number of autoimmune diseases when the condition is organ- or life-threatening. Examples are severe lupus nephritis presenting with renal failure, or ANCA vasculitis presenting with respiratory failure secondary to diffuse alveolar hemorrhage. Cyclophosphamide was previously a more widely used immunosuppressant, but less toxic medications have started to replace it. It is still used in advanced cases that have failed conventional therapies. Cyclophosphamide can be taken either orally or intravenously.

The side effects of cyclophosphamide are numerous, which limits its use to only the most life-threatening scenarios. Cyclophosphamide decreases cell division, so it also decreases the bone marrow's ability to produce cells, which can cause bone marrow suppression and decreased white blood cell, red blood cell, and platelet counts. Cyclophosphamide increases the patient's risk for infection and has other unique side effects, including *infertility* and *bladder cancer*.

Cyclophosphamide can decrease fertility in both women and men, dramatically decreasing its application to younger patients. If cyclophosphamide is required, fertility preservation needs to be discussed with patients prior to its implementation.

The incidence of bladder cancer is higher in patients who have used cyclophosphamide. Patients taking cyclophosphamide orally need to drink large amounts of water with the drug and also completely empty their bladder before going to bed, as this is thought to limit the exposure of the bladder to the medication.

## Targeted Therapy

The following drugs have changed the landscape in the treatment of rheumatologic diseases, ushering in a new era in which many patients are considered in full remission. Every year the pathophysiology of autoimmune diseases becomes better understood; each step in the understanding of these diseases often presents a new target for disease treatment. It's important to note that none of these drugs "cure" rheumatologic conditions. The goal is to continue using the medications and keep the patient in remission. A summary of the targeted therapies is presented in **Figure 2-7**.

*Tumor-necrosis factor (TNF) inhibitors* were the first targeted therapy for rheumatoid arthritis. TNF is a cytokine that is found in abundance in the synovium of patients with active rheumatoid arthritis. Multiple TNF inhibitors exist. They are administered by either subcutaneous injection or infusion. They include *infliximab (Remicade), adalimumab (Humira), etanercept (Enbrel), certolizumab pegol (Cimzia)*, and *golimumab (Simponi)*.

Since TNF is important for the functioning of the immune system, TNF inhibitors increase the risk of infections. The vast majority of TNF inhibitor-induced infections are minor, such as upper respiratory tract infections that may become more frequent and prolonged compared to patients not on TNF inhibitors. There is also a greater risk of serious infections, such as pneumonia. Rare side effects, such as a demyelinating process similar to multiple sclerosis, can be seen with TNF inhibitors. These usually are reversible on stopping the drug. A controversial side effect is an increased risk of malignancy, especially lymphoma. At the time of this writing, it is still unclear whether this slightly increased risk of lymphoma is due to the TNF inhibitor or the underlying autoimmune disease. There is some evidence of TNF inhibitors exacerbating heart failure, so these meds are generally avoided in patients with heart failure.

*Interleukin (IL) inhibitors.* Interleukins are a complex family of cytokines that are pivotal in a variety of autoimmune diseases. Individual interleukins play different roles in different diseases, so it is critical to know which disease is being treated before employing these medications.

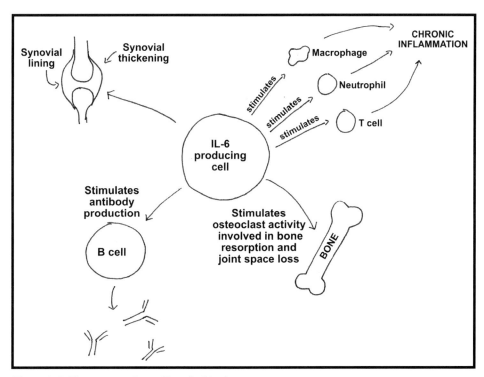

*Figure 2-5* *The many actions of interleukin-6.*

*Interleukin-1 inhibitors* were originally approved for the treatment of rheumatoid arthritis (RA), but their efficacy in treating RA appears to be less than other targeted therapies. It was later discovered that interleukin-1 is critical in autoinflammatory conditions, such as Familial Mediterranean Fever (FMF) and adult onset Still's disease (see Chapter 8, Autoinflammatory Disease). Interleukin-1 inhibitors have been used successfully in the treatment of crystalline disease (gout and pseudogout) and pericarditis. Interleukin-1 inhibitors include *anakinra (Kineret)*, *canakinumab (Ilaris)*, and *rilonacept (Arcalyst)*.

Side effects of IL-1 inhibition include immunosuppression, neutropenia, and injection site irritation.

*Interleukin-5.* Among its many actions, interleukin-5 stimulates eosinophil production. Blocking interleukin-5 thus dramatically decreases the production of eosinophils, which is clinically relevant in a number of allergic conditions, such as asthma and also in *Eosinophilic Granulomatosis with Polyangiitis (EGPA)* (see Chapter 13, Vasculitis). *Mepolizumab (Nucala)* is an interleukin-5 inhibitor.

Side effects of mepolizumab include headaches, injection site reactions, and increased risk of infections.

*Interleukin-6* appears to play a pivotal role in multiple diseases, prominently in rheumatoid arthritis and Giant Cell Arteritis (see Chapter 13, Vasculitis). The pathophysiology of interleukin-6's role in rheumatoid arthritis is multifactorial and involves stimulation of inflammation (macrophages, neutrophils, and T cells), stimulation of B cells to produce antibodies, stimulation of endothelial cells to grow into a pannus (see Chapter 3, Rheumatoid Arthritis), and stimulation of bone resorption and joint destruction (**Fig. 2-5**). Interleukin-6 inhibitors include *tocilizumab (Actemra)* and *sarilumab (Kevzara).*

*Interleukin-17* appears important in the pathogenesis of spondyloarthritis, including ankylosing spondylitis. Interleukin-17 also plays an important role in protecting from fungal organisms, so blocking this pathway may lead to an increased risk of fungal infections (usually cutaneous). *Secukinumab (Cosentyx)* is an interleukin-17 inhibitor.

*Interleukin-12* and *interleukin-23* both share a specific protein (protein 40). When protein 40 is targeted, this blocks both interleukin-12 and interleukin-23. These interleukins have been associated with activity of spondyloarthritis and especially inflammatory bowel disease. *Ustekinumab (Stelara)* is a medication that blocks interleukins-12 and -23.

***T cell interference.*** As of this writing, *abatacept (Orencia)* is the only medication used in systemic autoimmune diseases that directly interferes with the function of T cells. For a T cell to be activated, it needs to be activated by an antigen-presenting cell, a cell that presents a piece of protein from a virus or bacteria to the T cell. This activation is accomplished in two steps:

Signal 1: Binding of specific receptors on the antigen-presenting cell
Signal 2: Binding of specific receptors on the T cell

Both of the above (Signals 1 and 2) have to be completed for the T cell to be activated. Abatacept works by interfering with the T cell's ability to be activated, by blocking the second signal on the antigen-presenting cell **(Fig. 2-6)**. Abatacept is approved for the treatment of rheumatoid arthritis, psoriatic arthritis, and juvenile idiopathic arthritis.

*JAK/STAT inhibitors.* JAK/STAT is a signaling pathway used in a variety of inflammatory cytokines. If the pathway of these cytokines is blocked, then one medication can block a number of inflammatory cytokines. Considering multiple cytokines are blocked, it would be reasonable to conclude that patients on JAK/STAT inhibitors would be at higher risk of more side effects than other medications. So far this hasn't been the case, although patients on these medications do seem to be more prone to herpes zoster infections (shingles). Many trials are currently underway for a variety of JAK/STAT inhibitors. The most common currently used JAK/STAT inhibitor is *tofacitinib (Xeljanz)*, used to treat rheumatoid arthritis and psoriatic arthritis. JAK/STAT inhibitors are also the only targeted therapy that can be taken orally.

*B cell depleting therapies* were originally designed to treat B cell non-Hodgkin lymphoma. *Rituximab* is the B cell depleting agent most widely used in treating autoimmune diseases. Rituximab acts by binding to the protein receptor CD20, which resides on many types of B cells. This binding triggers activation of the immune system, which leads to death of the B cell. When the B cells are depleted, antibody production decreases dramatically. The medication usually has an effect for 6 months, and, depending on the disease being treated, the drug is reintroduced every 6 months. Dramatically decreasing the amount of B cells and antibodies in the blood of patients seems like it would have profound effects on the immune system and the ability of the patient to fight off infections. Most patients, though, do very well on B cell depleting agents. Currently, Rituximab is most often used in initiating treatment in ANCA vasculitis (see Chapter 13, Vasculitis) and is often used to treat patients with rheumatoid arthritis who have failed DMARD and anti-TNF therapy.

Like all immunosuppressive therapies, B cell depletion increases the risk of infections. A rare but serious complication of rituximab therapy is *progressive multifocal leukoencephalopathy*, a brain infection caused by the JC virus. There is no treatment for this condition, and it can be fatal. This side effect is rare, but patients need to know about it before therapy is begun with B cell depleting agents.

*Belimumab*, a medication in the category of B cell depletion, is much less potent than rituximab. It acts by blocking factors that help B cells survive, called *BLyS* and *BAFF*. These B cell survival factors may be elevated, particularly in systemic lupus erythematosus, and are thought to be involved in B cells surviving and producing harmful antibodies. By blocking these factors, B cells are more likely to undergo *apoptosis* (normal cell death). As of this writing, the only disease for which belimumab has been shown to be effective is systemic lupus erythematosus with non-renal involvement.

## Other Immunosuppressive Drugs

*Intravenous Immunoglobulin (IVIG).* Immunoglobulin is another word for *antibody*, the protein produced by B cells for immune memory. Originally, intravenous immunoglobulin was used in patients who had certain immunodeficiencies, such as B cell deficiency, and thus

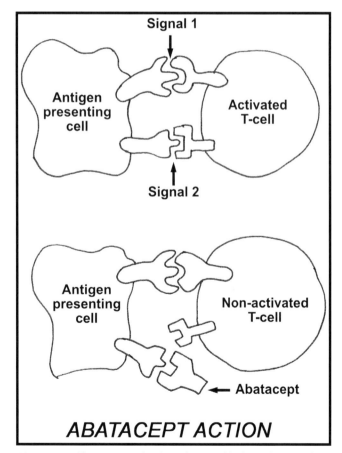

*Figure 2-6 Abatacept mechanism of action: blocking the second signal, preventing T-cell activation.*

lacked antibodies, making the patient infection-prone and unable to develop long-term memory against infection. IVIG in higher doses was later discovered to confer an anti-inflammatory effect and could be used to treat patients with a variety of autoimmune conditions, including inflammatory myopathy and myasthenia gravis. The mechanism of action of how intravenous immune globulin confers this benefit to autoimmune conditions is not clear.

One of the unique aspects of intravenous immunoglobulin is that it is one of the only medications rheumatologists give that does not suppress the immune system.

*Apremilast (Otezla)* is used to treat psoriasis and psoriatic arthritis. Apremilast works by blocking phosphodiesterase 4 (PGE4), which is needed for the production of TNF.

*Dapsone* is primarily used as an antibiotic, but a separate mechanism of action occurs that decreases neutrophil function. Dapsone is mostly used for cutaneous involvement in autoimmune diseases. It has other anti-inflammatory effects that are not well understood. Importantly, patients on dapsone need to be evaluated for glucose-6-phosphate dehydrogenase deficiency

(G-6-PD); a patient deficient in this enzyme is at risk of developing hemolytic anemia while on dapsone.

*Colchicine* is most often used by rheumatologists to rapidly decrease inflammation caused by crystalline diseases, such as gout and pseudogout. Colchicine is thought to decrease the ability of neutrophils to migrate to areas of inflammation, such as the joint. It is usually well tolerated as long as patients have normal renal function. Colchicine can cause bone marrow suppression in patients with poor renal function.

# Overview of Immunosuppressive Medication in Autoimmune Diseases

Few autoimmune diseases have a set treatment algorithm when initiating treatment. A good example is rheumatoid arthritis, probably the best studied of all the diseases. It has a variety of approved medications. However, besides the first two steps (first initiate a DMARD therapy such as methotrexate; if this does not control the disease, then use a TNF inhibitor), if the disease is still not controlled, then you can use any of the other approved medications. The point is, few of the

| FIGURE 2-7 TARGETED IMMUNE THERAPIES | | | | |
|---|---|---|---|---|
| | **Mechanism of Action** | **Administration** | **Safety Surveillance** | **Contraindications** |
| **TNF inhibitors** | Block TNF | IV or subcutaneous | CMP every 3 months | History of melanoma, heart failure, chronic infection |
| **Interleukin-1 inhibitor** | Blocks IL-1 | subcutaneous | CBC monthly | Chronic infections |
| **Interleukin-5 inhibitor** | Blocks IL-5 | subcutaneous | | Acute asthma attack, chronic infection |
| **Interleukin-6 inhibitor** | Blocks IL-6 | IV or subcutaneous | CBC, CMP and lipids every 3 months | Severe anemia, elevated liver enzymes, diverticulitis, chronic infection |
| **Interleukin-17 inhibitor** | Blocks IL-17 | subcutaneous | CMP every 3 months | Chronic infection |
| **Interleukin-12/23 inhibitor** | Blocks IL-12/23 | subcutaneous | | Chronic infection |
| **T cell inhibitor** | Blocks 2nd signal for T cell activation | IV or subcutaneous | | Chronic infection, COPD |
| **JAK/STAT inhibitor** | Blocks the signaling of multiple cytokines | oral | CBC and CMP every 3 months | Diverticulitis, severe anemia |
| **Rituximab** | Blocks CD20, which inhibits production of B cells | IV | | Chronic infection |
| **Belimumab** | Blocks B cell survival factors BLyS and BAFF | IV | | Chronic infection |

newer medications have been studied in comparative trials, so it is difficult to know which of the newer drugs is superior to the others. Each family of medications has unique side effects and routes of administration that should be discussed with the patient, and a shared decision made. The rarer diseases, such as polyarteritis nodosa and relapsing polychondritis, only have small, non-randomized studies to guide treatment. Only a few rheumatologic diseases, such as rheumatoid arthritis, spondyloarthritis and ANCA vasculitis, have randomized controlled trials to help guide therapy.

Rheumatology is often confusing to physicians outside the specialty because they see a variety of medications being utilized on patients, and it is difficult to understand why individual medications were selected over others. In reality, it was most likely a shared decision-making process between the patient and physician that selected the medication. **Figure 2-8** summarizes the many medications used in rheumatology and the diseases they are used for. This table will change rapidly over the years.

| FIGURE 2-8 IMMUNOSUPPRESSIVE DRUGS IN AUTOIMMUNE DISEASES | | | | | | | | |
|---|---|---|---|---|---|---|---|---|
| | Rheumatoid Arthritis | SpA (psoriatic arthritis, IBD associated arthritis) | Juvenile Idiopathic Arthritis (JIA) | SLE | Autoinflammatory Conditions (Familial Mediterranean Fever, Systemic JIA) | Inflammatory Myopathy | Giant Cell Arteritis | ANCA Vasculitis |
| DMARDs | YES | X (not ankylosing spondylitis) | YES | YES (MMF in SLE related renal disease) | YES | X | Mildly beneficial | YES (methotrexate for induction of mild disease, Azathioprine for maintenance therapy) |
| TNF inhibitor | YES | YES | YES | | ? | | | |
| Interleukin-1 | YES | | | | YES | | | |
| Interleukin-5 | | | | | | | | YES (EGPA) |
| Interleukin-6 | YES | | YES | | YES (Systemic JIA) | ? | YES | |
| Interleukin-12/23 | | YES | | | | | | |
| Interleukin-17 | | YES | | | | | | |
| T cells inhibitor (abatacept) | YES | YES | YES | | | | ? | |
| JAK/STAT inhibitor | YES | YES | YES | YES | ? | | | |
| PGE4 inhibitor | | YES | | | | | | |
| Belimumab | | | | YES | | | | |
| Rituximab | YES | | ? | ? | | | | YES |
| Cyclophos-phamide | | | | YES | | | | YES |

# Part II. Inflammatory Arthritis

The following three chapters review three diseases with a primary autoimmune inflammatory arthritis: *Rheumatoid Arthritis (RA), Spondyloarthritis (SpA), and Systemic Lupus Erythematosus (SLE)*. Yes, there are other systemic autoimmune diseases that present with inflammatory arthritis, but these three more commonly present with inflammatory arthritis as the primary complaint.

# 3

# *Rheumatoid Arthritis*

*Rheumatoid Arthritis (RA)* is a classic autoimmune inflammatory arthritis that affects people of all ages. RA is one of the more common autoimmune diseases with a prevalence ranging from 0.6-1.0% of the population. RA develops in a wide age range with peak incidence at 50-60 years but can occur from teenagers to people in their 80's. We do not know why this disease occurs. The overall pathophysiology of RA is incompletely understood but seems to be driven by high amounts of tumor necrosis factor (TNF), interleukin-1, and interleukin-6 within the joint space.

## History in Rheumatoid Arthritis

RA is classically a symmetric polyarticular inflammatory arthritis **(Fig. 3-1).** It presents over weeks to months with progressive joint pain, swelling, and stiffness. The patient describes pain, swelling, and stiffness on arising in the morning; it takes an hour or more to start feeling improvement in the joints although the pain may persist. Within the first few weeks of disease onset, the joint involvement may be unilateral, but will usually become bilateral within months.

Consider RA whenever someone presents with *symmetric polyarticular* inflammatory arthritis. Let's break that down:

- *Symmetric:* If a joint is involved (say the wrist), it's going to be both left and right wrists.

- *Polyarticular*: This means 5 or more joints, which is pretty easy to happen if the metacarpal phalangeal joints (MCPs) of both hands are involved.

- *Inflammatory:* The immune system activation causes swollen, painful joints that usually get better the more the person uses them. The symptoms usually come on gradually over weeks or months. Nearly all patients with rheumatoid arthritis will have morning stiffness in the affected joints, lasting for more than 1 hour. As with other autoimmune inflammatory arthritis, the pain of rheumatoid arthritis (especially early in the disease) improves with activity.

These are the joints to look for:

- MCPs **(Fig. 3-2)**, proximal interphalangeal joints (PIPs), wrists, and metatarsophalangeal joints (MTPs), but RA can affect many other joints**.**

- The joint pain and swelling can also start in the feet and ankles. This is important, because when x-rays are performed, the 5th toe metatarsal phalangeal joint is often the first joint to develop erosions (joint damage seen on x-rays).

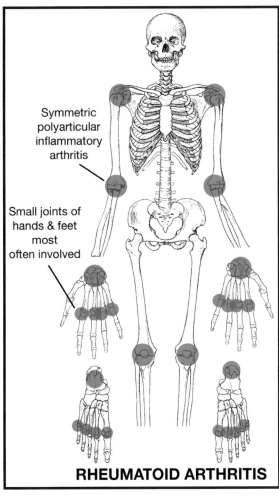

Figure 3-1 *Symmetric polyarticular inflammatory arthritis.*

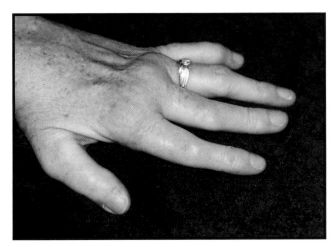

Figure 3-2 *Metacarpal phalangeal joint (MCP) swelling in a patient with RA. Image courtesy of the American College of Rheumatology.*

Unusual joints for RA:

- Distal interphalangeal joints (DIPs). DIP involvement is unusual for RA and is more consistent with spondyloarthritis and osteoarthritis, which are discussed later.
- Spinal involvement in RA is unusual except for the cervical spine, which is discussed later. Spinal involvement is more classic for spondyloarthritis.

## Physical Exam in Rheumatoid Arthritis

With active disease you'll note some *warmth* and *puffiness* to the joint and possibly some *erythema*; this is the clinical picture of *synovitis*.

When the patient makes a fist, the ridges of the MCPs will no longer be well defined **(Fig. 1-6)**.

Pain is elicited with pressing on the affected joints as well as flexion and extension of the joints.

In long-standing RA you might find permanent deformities of the hands from joint destruction, as well as ligament laxity from chronic inflammation around the ligaments. The laxity around the ligaments can make the joints hyperextend (*swan neck deformity*) (**Figs. 3-3, 3-4**). In most cases, the destruction and deformity happen over months to years of chronic inflammation. Joint destruction of the MCPs can cause the fingers to deviate to the ulnar side (*ulnar deviation*). In RA,

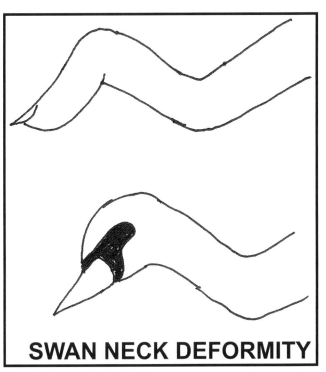

Figure 3-3 *Comparing the swan neck deformity of a finger with advanced rheumatoid arthritis to an actual swan neck.*

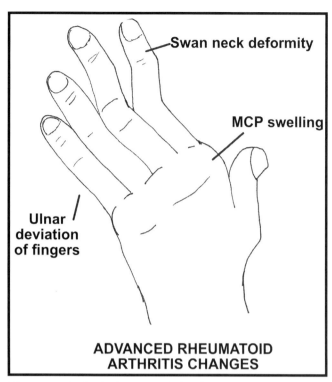

Swan neck deformity

MCP swelling

Ulnar deviation of fingers

**ADVANCED RHEUMATOID ARTHRITIS CHANGES**

*Figure 3-4* *Multiple changes in the hands in a patient with advanced rheumatoid arthritis.*

the examiner cannot grasp the fingers and straighten out ulnar deviation as you can in other autoimmune conditions (systemic lupus erythematosus).

## Extra-articular Manifestations of RA

RA isn't always confined just to the joints. You may see the following extra-articular manifestations when a patient has active, difficult-to-control disease over a long period of time:

*Constitutional.* Like most inflammatory conditions, whenever the disease is active, the patients will often experience fatigue and occasional fevers.

*Rheumatoid nodules.* These more commonly occur in seropositive patients. For unknown reasons, patients can develop painless or painful skin nodules, usually in areas where the skin has contacted hard surfaces (e.g. at the elbows). The nodules usually don't require specific treatment, but if they limit joint movement, they can be injected with steroid, which can sometimes shrink them. Another option is to surgically remove the nodules.

*Lung disease.* Interstitial fibrosis, pulmonary nodules, and organizing pneumonia (pneumonia caused by chronic inflammation and not infection) can all occur in patients with RA.

*Neck instability (atlantoaxial instability).* Atlantoaxial instability is an articular component of RA, but it's rare in the age of targeted therapy. Atlantoaxial instability refers to excessive movement between parts of the neck vertebrae, namely the atlas (C1) and axis (C2). This can cause spinal cord compression, leading to paralysis. This instability becomes especially important in rheumatoid arthritis patients undergoing intubation for surgery, since the neck will be manipulated, with possible subsequent spinal cord compression. Patients with rheumatoid arthritis should have x-rays of the neck prior to surgery, which can detect excessive laxity.

*Felty's Syndrome* is a rare complication of rheumatoid arthritis where the patient develops a low white blood cell count, particularly low neutrophils (neutropenia) as well as splenomegaly on abdominal imaging. It's unclear why this occurs in patients with uncontrolled rheumatoid arthritis. Treating the underlying rheumatoid arthritis may help the neutropenia.

## Laboratory Findings in Rheumatoid Arthritis

Two blood markers are important for the diagnosis of rheumatoid arthritis:

- *Rheumatoid factor (RF)* is a sensitive but less specific blood test for rheumatoid arthritis.
- *Anti-Cyclic citrullinated peptide (CCP)* is a more specific test.

The blood in most patients with RA will be positive for RF or CCP or both. When a patient has an inflammatory arthritis along with either RF or CCP positivity, this is called *seropositive RA.* If a patient has a symmetric polyarticular inflammatory arthritis with negative RF and negative CCP, and other causes have been ruled out (see Chapter 7, Infectious Causes of Inflammatory Joint Pain), this is called *seronegative rheumatoid arthritis.* This is an important prognostic distinction, as patients who are seropositive are at increased risk for more rapid progression compared to patients with seronegative rheumatoid arthritis.

## Imaging Findings in Rheumatoid Arthritis

*Erosions on x-ray.* Erosions are areas on the bony surface of the joint that have been destroyed by chronic inflammation. They can be appreciated on x-ray, appearing like small scoops taken out of the bone **(Fig. 3-5)**. In early RA, x-ray of the hands and feet may be normal. One of the goals of treatment is to prevent erosions from occurring.

Remember an x-ray only shows the bony changes occurring in autoimmune disease like rheumatoid arthritis. Synovial inflammation will not be visible on an x-ray image **(Fig. 3-6)**.

*Bone loss.* Osteopenia (decreased bone density) is common in patients with RA. You can see it on x-rays of the hands because there will be less bone density around the joints affected by the disease (*peri-articular osteopenia*).

More advanced imaging studies, such as Magnetic Resonance Imaging (MRI) and Ultrasound (US), are better for showing changes in the soft tissue around the joint and can demonstrate evidence of synovitis.

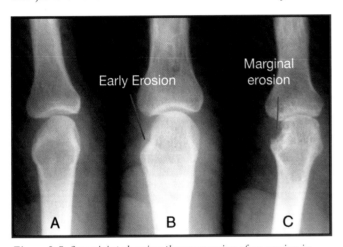

*Figure 3-5 Same joint showing the progression of an erosion in a patient with rheumatoid arthritis. A: no erosion yet. B: early erosion. C: marginal erosion. Notice that the bone near the joint appears slightly less dense (white), even in early disease (peri-articular osteopenia).*

MRI and US are most often used in times of clinical uncertainty about the diagnosis, and can provide more objective evidence of joint inflammation.

## Treatment of Rheumatoid Arthritis

The good news about RA is that we have many medications to control it, making many of the extra-articular manifestations less common. The treatment of RA has greatly changed in the last few decades. Every year there seems to be a new RA drug with a new mechanism of action.

*Rapid treatment.* To rapidly reduce swelling and pain, NSAIDs and glucocorticoids can be initiated. Response to glucocorticoids and NSAIDs is also helpful diagnostically; if no improvement is seen in the patient's pain, RA is less likely the cause of the joint pain.

*Long-term management.* The goal of long-term therapy is use of an immunosuppressing agent that is well tolerated, controls the symptoms of RA, and prevents disease progression. Classically, methotrexate is the first line drug; this will control the disease by itself about 30% of the time. If methotrexate doesn't completely control the disease, a targeted/biologic therapy or another DMARD agent is added to the methotrexate. There are multiple different types of biologic and non-biologic therapies that treat RA very well. (See Chapter 2, The Immune System and Treatment in Rheumatology, for more details.)

*Long-term prognosis of RA.* In modern times, the prognosis of RA is overall good. Like other autoimmune diseases, RA cannot be cured, but it can be treated to the point of preventing pain and subsequent joint

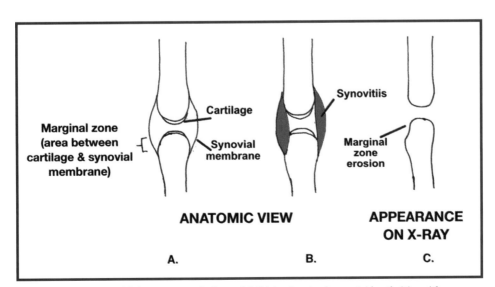

*Figure 3-6 A. Normal joint anatomy. B. Synovial thickening in rheumatoid arthritis, with synovitis. C. The chronic synovial thickening eventually erodes into the bone, seen on x-ray as a marginal zone erosion.*

destruction. The treatment for RA is rapidly evolving, with new medications continually arising. If untreated, RA can cause significant disability, with depression and loss of employment. Before the discovery of biologic medications, patients commonly had severe joint deformities and joint destruction in the hands from years of chronic joint inflammation.

## Other Rheumatoid Arthritis-like Entities

*Palindromic rheumatoid arthritis* looks just like rheumatoid arthritis, but the pain and swelling are intermittent instead of daily. Usually rheumatoid arthritis presents with daily pain and swelling, but palindromic rheumatoid arthritis may behave more like crystalline disease (gout, pseudogout) in that the hand pain and swelling may present for a few days, then resolve. The best way to prove it's not gout is to draw fluid from the inflamed joints and evaluate for crystals; many of these patients will have positive rheumatoid factor and positive anti-CCP, which help establish the diagnosis. A large fraction of palindromic rheumatoid arthritis cases progress into "regular rheumatoid arthritis," but the overall prognosis is very good, usually requiring less aggressive medication.

*Remitting seronegative symmetrical synovitis with pitting edema* is a difficult disease to remember, so just remember RS3PE. RS3PE presents with hand swelling similar to rheumatoid arthritis, but instead of just the joints, the entire hand is often swollen, making the hands look like baseball gloves. RS3PE often has pitting edema, meaning the examiner can push into the back of the patient's hand and it will leave an indentation; rheumatoid arthritis swelling is usually confined to the joints, and the swelling is non-pitting. RS3PE usually resolves rapidly with minimal steroid treatment. When evaluating a patient with RS3PE, rule out underlying malignancy; RS3PE is highly associated with cancer, especially hematologic malignancies.

## CASES

1. HISTORY: A 32-year-old woman with no significant past medical history presents with joint pain and swelling in eight of her MCPs, wrists bilaterally, and four of her MTPs. The joint pain has been worsening for the past 5 months. She notes the pain as a dull ache with associated stiffness. She feels it's much worse in the morning and improves with activity throughout the day.

   LABORATORY: Her blood tests are rheumatoid factor and anti-cyclic citrullinated peptide positive.

   TREATMENT: This patient's clinical presentation and blood work are consistent with seropositive rheumatoid arthritis. Initial treatment can include glucocorticoids (prednisone 20 mg) and NSAIDs (ibuprofen) to quickly help the joint pain. For long-term management, methotrexate can be started at 15 mg once a week along with supplementary folic acid daily to limit the side effects of methotrexate. Methotrexate will take 2-3 months to show clinical efficacy, so the patient can be continued on a slow taper of prednisone and ibuprofen while methotrexate begins to work. Make sure to have the patient screened for tuberculosis and hepatitis B and C prior to initiating immunosuppressive medication.

2. HISTORY: The same patient presents back to your office 3 months later. She feels the prednisone has completely taken away her pain. She can't seem to taper the prednisone down below 10 mg without worsening pain and swelling of her MCPs.

   TREATMENT: At this point you have given the methotrexate 3 months to start working, but her disease is still not controlled without the use of a moderate amount of prednisone. Prednisone isn't a good long-term option because of the numerous side effects of prolonged steroid use, so more aggressive management is needed. The options at this point would be to add an additional disease-modifying anti-rheumatic drug (*DMARD*) such as *sulfasalazine*, or add a tumor necrosis factor inhibitor such as *adalimumab*. TNF inhibitors are usually the first biologic used after failure of DMARD therapy. This is not because they are more efficacious than other biologics but because they have been around longer, and we have more data for their use. If a TNF inhibitor is not efficacious within 2-3 months, then the patient can either be switched to another TNF inhibitor or changed to a drug with a completely different mechanism of action.

# 4

# Spondyloarthritis (SpA)

*Spondyloarthritis (SpA)* is an umbrella term for four different diseases that overlap with one another. The prevalence of SpA ranges greatly, from 0.2-1.2% of the population depending on the part of the world. SpA usually presents earlier in life (20-30 years of age) but later is also possible. The word *spondyloarthritis* refers to joint inflammation of the spine, which is appropriate as all four diseases in this category can have spinal involvement (but many times they do not). The four diseases of SpA are

- *Ankylosing spondylitis*
- *Inflammatory bowel disease associated arthritis*
- *Psoriatic arthritis*
- *Reactive arthritis* (previously called *Reiter's syndrome*)

These diseases are all classified under SpA because their presentations can overlap with one another and have similar genetic predispositions (HLA-B27). By "overlapping," I mean that a patient with one SpA disease can later develop components of another SpA disease. For example, classic ankylosing spondylitis has inflammatory back pain, while psoriatic arthritis is psoriasis with an inflammatory arthritis in the hands. These diseases can overlap since the patient with psoriatic arthritis can have hand pain as well as inflammatory back pain (psoriatic arthritis with axial involvement). Sometimes you may have difficulty knowing exactly what to call the disease, but the important thing is recognizing that the patient has SpA.

We don't know why this disease occurs, but like other autoimmune diseases, it's likely a combination of genetic predisposition and an environmental trigger. As of this writing, the main contributors to inflammation in this disease appear to be cyclooxygenase (COX), tumor necrosis factor alpha (TNF alpha), interleukin-17 and interleukin-23.

## Ankylosing Spondylitis (AS)

*Ankylosing spondylitis* is the spondyloarthritis you will probably see most on internal medicine exams, such as the Internal Medicine boards. This disease primarily involves the lower back and sacroiliac (SI) joints in young patients and causes inflammatory back pain. You'll often see patients with back pain in your office, but what is particular about AS patients is they are young, usually in their 20's. We normally associate back pain with an older age group, so a young patient with non-traumatic, chronic back pain should set off alarm bells.

Let's break down the name of the disease. "Ankylosing" means that a joint becomes fused. The space between the joint disappears; the bone bridges from one end to another. As you can imagine, when ankylosis occurs, you no longer have the same mobility. "Spondylitis" means inflammation of the bones of the spine. So, ankylosing spondylitis refers to the joints of the back fusing after chronic back inflammation.

This inflammation and fusion occur mostly in the sacroiliac joints of the pelvis and the lumbar spine.

Therefore, low back pain and stiffness are usually the predominant symptoms. Importantly, fusion of the joints is a late finding. If you see the patients within the first months or years of their symptoms, they probably won't have fused joints on imaging. Before non-steroidal anti-inflammatory medications and newer biologic therapies, most of these patients would have progressed to fused joints and severely restricted back mobility.

## Inflammatory Bowel Disease-Associated Arthritis

If you see a young patient for joint pain with a history of Crohn's disease or ulcerative colitis, then *IBD-associated arthritis* should be high on your differential. Inflammatory bowel diseases (Crohn's and ulcerative colitis) are associated with inflammatory arthritis, and they fit into the SpA category. The patient can present with axial involvement, peripheral involvement, or both. The inflammatory joint pain symptoms can coincide with the Inflammatory Bowel Disease (IBD) symptoms, but, strangely, more often than not the joint pain can flare independently of the IBD symptoms.

## Psoriatic Arthritis

As the name suggests, *psoriatic arthritis* is an inflammatory arthritis in patients with psoriasis. Psoriasis is a skin condition that causes small to large plaque-like lesions on elbows, knees, and other extensor surfaces. Like IBD, most patients with psoriasis do not have inflammatory arthritis, but when you see a patient with a history of psoriasis presenting with joint pain, this is something you should think about. To make life more difficult, a minority of patients with psoriatic arthritis initially present with inflammatory arthritis, then develop psoriasis months to years later, making the initial diagnosis not so straightforward. *Peripheral SpA* sometimes refers to psoriatic arthritis without psoriasis. The word *peripheral* is important here as it stresses that the symptoms are confined to peripheral joints, and not axial involvement (inflammatory back pain).

Psoriatic arthritis, more so than the other SpAs, may present with a polyarticular, symmetric inflammatory arthritis (more often than an oligoarticular, asymmetric inflammatory arthritis). It is more commonly polyarticular because the distal interphalangeal joints (DIPs) are usually involved, which can add up quickly! In SpA, the medium to large joints are usually asymmetric, but if the small joints (fingers) become involved, the fingers are symmetric and polyarticular

(the DIPs of most fingers on both left and right hand). Classically, a patient with psoriatic arthritis presents with swollen, warm, and painful distal finger joints. The patient may also notice multiple little pits in the nails. Usually, the more the patients use their fingers, the better they feel. They usually feel stiff for more than 1 hour in the morning.

## Reactive Arthritis

*Reactive arthritis* is an inflammatory arthritic reaction to a recent infection, most commonly an upper respiratory tract infection or diarrheal illness. It's thought that in genetically predisposed individuals, the immune system overreacts to these infections and starts attacking the joints as well as other organ systems. This is the disease you heard about in medical school when people said, "Can't see (conjunctivitis or uveitis), can't pee (urethritis), can't climb a tree (inflammatory arthritis)." Reactive arthritis is the rarest of the SpA diseases, but it is also associated with the genetic marker HLA-B27. Classically, patients complain of a severe diarrheal illness that preceded the joint pain by a few weeks or even months. The joint pain is more commonly *oligoarticular* (2-4 joints) and asymmetric in the medium and large joints. For unknown reasons, the involved joints are more likely in the lower extremities. A patient may present with a swollen left knee, a swollen right ankle, and possibly a swollen 4th right toe (*dactylitis*).

We don't know why reactive arthritis happens; it seems more common after certain infections. Of note, the vast majority of patients infected with these organisms will not develop a reactive arthritis. The following are the most common infections associated with subsequent reactive arthritis **(Fig. 4-1)**.

### Diagnosis of Reactive Arthritis

When considering the diagnosis of reactive arthritis, it helps to find evidence of a preceding infection with one of the more common organisms. If the patient has painful urination or discharge from the penis

| FIGURE 4-1 COMMON INFECTIONS ASSOCIATED WITH SUBSEQUENT REACTIVE ARTHRITIS | |
|---|---|
| **Infectious Organism** | **Infection** |
| Chlamydia trachomatis | Urethritis |
| Chlamydia pneumoniae | Pneumonia |
| Yersinia, Campylobacter, Salmonella, Shigella, E. Coli, Clostridium difficile | Diarrhea |

or vagina (possible urethritis), send the urine for a chlamydia test. If the patient continues to have active diarrhea, send a stool culture to try and identify the causal organism.

## Treatment of Reactive Arthritis

Treatment for reactive arthritis differs from other types of SpA because the duration of reactive arthritis may be self-limited; whereas ankylosing spondylitis, IBD associated arthritis, and psoriatic arthritis are much more likely to be chronic. A reasonable question: If the inflammatory arthritis is secondary to an infection, will the inflammatory arthritis go away if you treat the infection? Probably not right away. In patients with genitourinary tract infections such as chlamydia, treat both the patient and sexual partner. Treatment of enteric organisms (diarrhea) is less indicated, as most of the time these illnesses are self-limited. There aren't any data to suggest that prompt treatment of these infections decreases the risk of developing reactive arthritis; again, the vast majority of patients with these infections will not develop reactive arthritis.

So, besides antibiotics, what do you do about the swollen joints? The first-line treatment is non-steroidal anti-inflammatory drugs (NSAIDs) to help with the pain and swelling. Usually, reactive arthritis is self-limited and the NSAIDs will be enough to get them over the disease.

If joint pain and inflammation continue for more than 6 months and cannot be controlled with NSAIDs, then the patient will most likely require a disease-modifying anti-rheumatic drug (DMARD) and even possibly an anti-TNF medication to control the disease.

# History in Spondyloarthritis (SpA)

Considering that the category of SpA includes multiple diseases that can overlap, it's difficult to explain how SpA presents; the presentation can vary greatly from one patient to another. It's easier to explain different ways in which SpA can affect different body parts, so if you see one of the following, you should consider SpA in the differential.

*Asymmetric oligoarticular inflammatory arthritis (medium and large joints).*

- *Asymmetric* means that if one joint is swollen, the contralateral joint is not. For example, if the left wrist is swollen, the right wrist is not. A typical presentation of asymmetric joint disease is left ankle swelling and right wrist swelling.
- *Oligoarticular* refers to the number of joints involved, between 2 and 4. *The caveat to this is, if the small joints are involved (DIPs), then the small joints*

*will be symmetric and polyarticular.* A patient may have the DIPs of all the digits on his right and left hand involved, as well as right wrist, left shoulder involvement. The medium and large joints are asymmetric.

- *Inflammatory Arthritis.* Like Rheumatoid Arthritis (RA), SpA is an autoimmune inflammatory arthritis, meaning the immune system causes joint swelling and pain that classically is worse in the morning and better with activity.

*Joints Involved.* When describing the joint involvement of a patient with SpA, it's important to categorize the patient as having axial involvement, peripheral involvement, or both. Axial involvement refers to the spine and pelvis; peripheral involvement is everywhere else, like the elbows, wrists and hands. An example is a patient with psoriatic arthritis with axial and peripheral involvement in the left wrist and left elbow. This is saying that the patient has inflammatory back pain but also inflammatory arthritis of peripheral joints. This is an important distinction to make; if the spine is involved then the management of the disease is different than if only the peripheral joints are involved. Management will be discussed in more detail at the end of the chapter.

*Axial involvement in SpA.* Spinal and pelvic involvement in SpA manifests as *inflammatory back pain*, which differs from ordinary mechanical back pain. Inflammatory back pain occurs when the immune system causes swelling and inflammation around the vertebral and sacroiliac (SI) joints of the back. New bone formation can occur along the spine **(Fig. 4-2)**. This typically presents as pain and stiffness first thing the morning, usually lasting over an hour, and improving with activity. In contrast, anatomic back pain, like a herniated disc or muscle strain, worsens with activity. Inflammatory back pain also often wakes the patient from sleep and usually improves with NSAID therapy. Especially consider inflammatory back pain in a younger patient presenting with back pain.

*Peripheral involvement in SpA.* Medium-sized joints: Classically SpA involves the medium joints, like the wrist, ankle and elbows and is oligoarticular (2-4 joints) asymmetric.

Small joints (DIPs): If a patient has hand involvement, the DIP joints are the most often affected. This can be confusing because if a patient with SpA has hand involvement, then the presentation can be symmetric and polyarticular. One of the ways to differentiate SpA from rheumatoid arthritis of the hand is the DIP involvement. RA involves the MCPs, and SpA involves the DIPs **(Fig. 4-3)**.

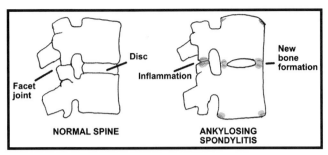

*Figure 4-2 Normal vertebra compared to vertebra with axial spondyloarthritis, displaying inflammation and new bone formation between the vertebrae, which can severely limit mobility.*

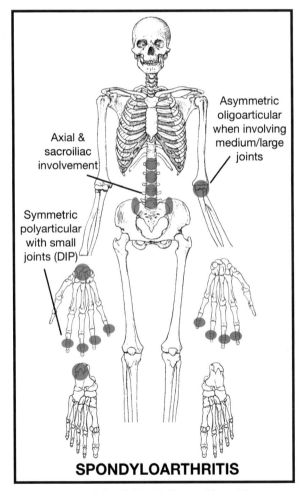

*Figure 4-3 Spondyloarthritis. Medium and large joints present with asymmetric oligoarticular inflammatory arthritis. Small joints like the hands present with symmetric polyarticular inflammatory arthritis in the distal interphalangeal joints. Axial (spinal) involvement can also occur.*

# Extra-Articular Manifestations of SpA

*Enthesitis.* Inflammation at the spot where the tendon or ligament inserts into the bone. This can happen in many different points in the body; a classic example is the insertion site of the Achilles tendon **(Fig. 4-4).**

*Dactylitis.* You'll notice this when a patient comes in with one large swollen finger or toe. The entire finger or toe will be swollen, not just the joint but also the soft tissue in between the joints (*sausage digit*).

*Tenosynovitis.* Inflammation around the tendon sheaths can occur in SpA, which makes it very painful for patients to use those particular muscles. You can test for tenosynovitis by placing resistance against the involved muscles, which will cause pain.

*Uveitis/conjunctivitis.* When evaluating a patient with suspected SpA, ask if there are any visual symptoms, such as eye redness, pain, or episodic blurry vision, which may indicate inflammation in the eye. If the patient has some of these symptoms, refer to an ophthalmologist to evaluate for uveitis, which, if present, raises suspicion for SpA.

*Psoriasis.* Psoriasis is a skin condition that causes thick, silvery-scaled red patches on the extensor surfaces of joints, such as the elbows or knees, but can appear anywhere on the body including the scalp.

*Inflammatory Bowel Disease.* Symptoms of IBD to inquire about include abdominal cramping, chronic diarrhea, or blood in the stool. If a patient has any of these gastrointestinal symptoms, gastroenterology should evaluate the patient with a colonoscopy to diagnose IBD.

# Physical Exam in Spondyloarthritis

The physical exam findings of SpA depend on the parts of the body involved.

*Skin.* Anyone suspected of having SpA should have a thorough skin exam to look for evidence of psoriasis. If an inflammatory arthritis is suspected and psoriasis is discovered on the body, the diagnosis of SpA is much more likely.

*Fingernails.* In patients with psoriasis and psoriatic arthritis, the fingernails may be thickened, with small dents as well (*nail pitting*).

*Joints.* Evaluate for swelling, pain with palpation, erythema around the DIPs of the fingers **(Fig. 4-5).**

*Tenosynovitis.* Tenosynovitis can be appreciated on exam by asking the patient to move a joint against resistance. For example, extensor tenosynovitis of the wrist can be detected by asking the patient to

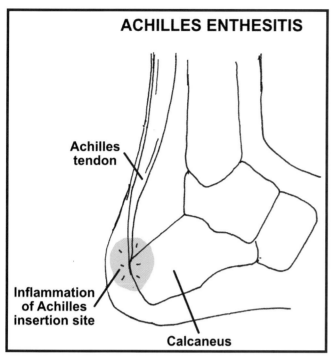

**Figure 4-4** *Achilles enthesitis. Inflammation at the Achilles tendon insertion into the calcaneus.*

dorsiflex the hand against resistance; if tenosynovitis is present, pain will shoot down the hand and across the wrist.

*Spinal exam.* The *Schober test* evaluates the mobility of the patient's lower back and can be used on patients with suspected ankylosing spondylitis. The test involves placing a mark on the skin of the patient 10 cm up the spine from the top of the iliac crest and then asking the patient to bend forward as far as possible while the examiner continues to hold the measuring tape at the spine at the base of the iliac crest. While the patient is fully bent forward, the measuring tape is re-applied to the spine and the measurer will see where the measuring tape lines up with the original 10 cm mark **(Figs. 4-6)**. Normally, the tape will line up at 15 cm with the original 10 cm mark, denoting a change in 5 cm with flexion of the spine. In a patient with ankylosing spondylitis, the measurement may only increase 1-2 cm, an abnormal Schober test. Keep in mind that the test will be normal in early disease and only become abnormal after significant damage has occurred.

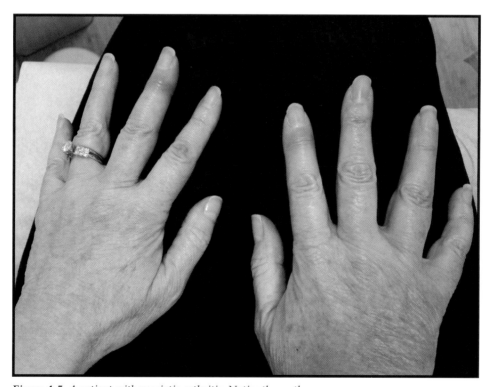

**Figure 4-5** *A patient with psoriatic arthritis. Notice the erythema of the distal interphalangeal joints.*

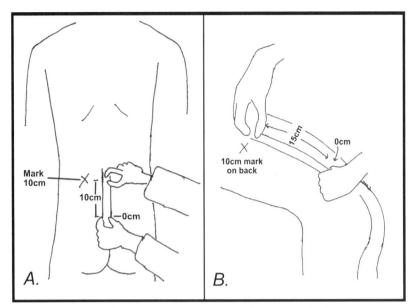

*Figure 4-6* *The Schober test. A. The examiner marks a zero at the base of the spine at the level of the pelvic brim, then measures up to 10 cm while the patient is standing upright. B. The patient bends forward while the examiner keeps a hand at the zero mark and then measures how much more length has been added with spine flexion to the previous 10 cm mark.*

## Laboratory and Imaging in Spondyloarthritis

*Blood tests.* No diagnostic blood tests for SpA are available; hence the commonly used name *seronegative spondyloarthropathy.* As with most rheumatologic diseases, when there is active inflammation, the patient's inflammatory markers (Erythrocyte Sedimentation Rate and C-reactive protein) will usually be elevated, but these changes are not specific for SpA.

*HLA-B27.* There is an association of HLA-B27 antigen with SpA, depending on the ethnic group (Caucasian patients with SpA are more commonly HLA-B27 positive than African Americans with SpA). Most patients with diagnosed SpA have a positive HLA-B27. However, HLA-B27 is not rare in the general population, and many people with HLA-B27 do not have SpA, making the testing for HLA-B27 nonspecific.

*X-ray.* X-rays can help in the workup of SpA, depending on what areas are involved. X-ray findings within the joint differ from what you would expect in rheumatoid arthritis. In SpA, erosions can be seen, but there may also be addition of bone around the joint (*syndesmophyte*).

*Hand.* A good example of the erosions and bone formation that occur in SpA is the *pencil-in-cup* changes of the DIPs typical of psoriatic arthritis. The pencil-in-cup deformity occurs when the distal end of the middle phalanx erodes down to a point, making the bone look like a pencil, and the proximal end of the distal phalanx can have bony proliferation that makes it look like a cup (**Figs. 4-7, 4-8**).

*Pelvis.* In advanced inflammatory back pain, changes can be seen in the sacroiliac joints on x-ray imaging. The SI joints may show erosions or joint fusion (**Figs. 4-9, 4-10**).

How are these diseases labeled? Considering that the diseases associated with SpA overlap, you may wonder how we name them. Usually, the first symptom the patient notices helps define the disease. A patient with psoriasis for a number of years who then develops inflammatory joint pain will be labeled as having psoriatic arthritis. If there is a multiple-year history of inflammatory bowel disease followed by inflammatory back pain, this is labeled IBD-associated arthritis. The important thing is recognizing that the patient has spondyloarthritis.

## Treatment of SpA

The following treatment discussion does not apply to reactive arthritis, which usually can be treated symptomatically without aggressive immunosuppressive medications.

As mentioned, it's important to note whether a patient has peripheral involvement, axial involvement, or both. The reason this distinction is important is that it changes therapy. If the patient presents with

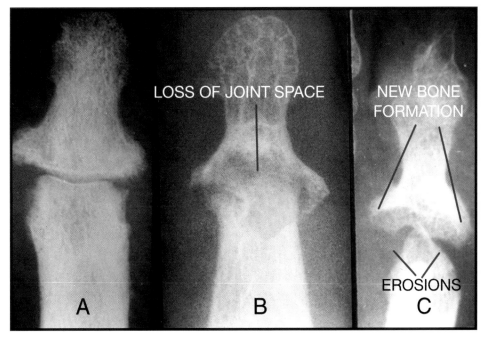

*Figure 4-7* *Distal interphalangeal joint of a patient with psoriatic arthritis, showing progressive x-ray changes over time, leading to a pencil-in-cup deformity. Image courtesy of the American College of Rheumatology.*

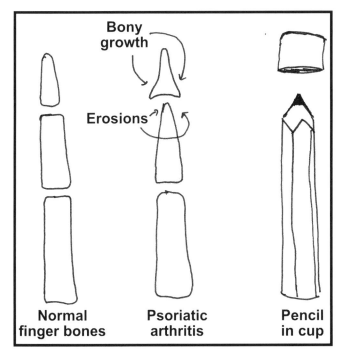

*Figure 4-8* *A normal finger bone compared with the pencil-in-cup deformity of psoriatic arthritis.*

no axial involvement, then starting with a Disease-Modifying Anti-Rheumatic Drug (DMARD) such as methotrexate is reasonable. If DMARD therapy does not control symptoms, then stepping up therapy with a biologic medication is reasonable. If the patient *has axial involvement*, then DMARD therapy will not benefit

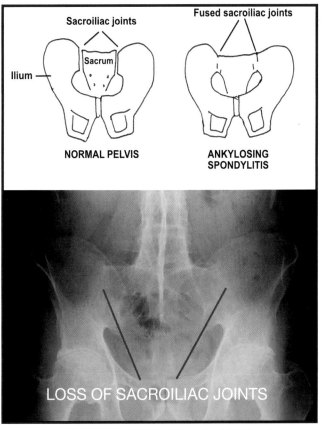

*Figure 4-9* *Ankylosing spondyloarthritis of pelvis. Drawing shows normal pelvis compared to one with advanced ankylosing spondylitis. Notice the fused sacroiliac joints. X-ray shows fusion of sacroiliac joint spaces.*

the patient's back symptoms; anti-TNF therapy can be initiated in these cases without having to use a DMARD first. The biologics that are currently used for different types of SpA are TNF inhibitors, IL-12/23 inhibitor, IL-17 inhibitor, phosphodiesterase 4 (PDE4) inhibitor, and the T cell inhibitor abatacept.

# Cases

1. HISTORY: A 32-year-old man presents with a history of chronic low back pain. He started noticing the pain about 10 years ago, intermittent at first but then developing into a more consistent dull aching pain and stiffness, much worse in the morning and progressively improving with more activity. The back pain sometimes awakens him at night. He usually takes an NSAID for the pain when it gets bad enough.

   PHYSICAL: On exam, you notice that he cannot fully rotate his neck left and right, and when he bends forward, he has limited range of motion. His Schober test shows a change of only 2 cm (normal is 5 cm or greater).

   LAB: X-ray of the pelvis shows erosions on the SI joint bilaterally.

   DIAGNOSIS: Ankylosing spondylitis.

   TREATMENT: On NSAIDs, the pain improves somewhat, but overall his symptoms are worsening. The concern is that he will continue to have decreased range of motion in his neck and back if treatment is not initiated. Disease-modifying anti-rheumatoid drugs (DMARDs) have not been shown to be efficacious in axial involvement of SpA. Since all his symptoms are axial, TNF inhibitors can be used to limit progression of the disease and help his pain without first using DMARD therapy. TNF inhibitors will help both axial and peripheral disease, whereas DMARD therapy will only help peripheral disease.

2. HISTORY: A 42-year-old man with a long-standing history of plaque psoriasis on his knees and elbows presents with pain at the tips of his fingers. In the last few months, he noticed an increasing dull ache in his distal interphalangeal joints (DIPs) as well as some redness and swelling. He notices improvement in the pain and swelling the more he moves his fingers, and by the afternoon he usually doesn't

have much pain. He has no history of red, painful eyes, and no history of chronic diarrhea or bloody stools. He also reports no history of lower back pain.

PHYSICAL: On exam, you notice mild warmth to the DIPs as well as some pain with palpation of the DIPs. The other hand joints are normal. He also has evidence of plaque psoriasis on his elbows and knees, which doesn't bother him very much.

DIAGNOSIS: His presentation is consistent with psoriatic arthritis.

TREATMENT: initial treatment should be aimed at decreasing the swelling and pain in the fingers, which can be done with DMARD therapy, e.g. methotrexate. This should be given for at least 3 months. If DMARD therapy does not improve the pain and swelling in his fingers, a TNF inhibitor can be used. If he has evidence of axial involvement (low back pain), do an x-ray of his SI joints and possibly an MRI. If evidence of inflammation is found in the lower back, give TNF inhibitors rather than DMARDs, which have not been shown to improve axial involvement in SpA.

3. HISTORY: A 22-year-old man presents with painful swelling of his left knee and right wrist, which started at the same time and has progressively worsened over the course of 3 weeks. He has a hard time using his right hand and walking because his left knee feels very stiff. He is recovering from a diarrheal illness that started one week ago. He also says he had left eye redness yesterday, but it resolved on its own. His labs are normal besides mildly elevated inflammatory markers; his ANA is negative.

   PHYSICAL: On exam, you note warmth in his left knee and right hand with minimal swelling and no effusion. The two joints are tender to touch. His sclera is currently white with no evidence of redness.

   DIAGNOSIS: This is most likely a reactive arthritis. The previous eye redness was likely either conjunctivitis or uveitis, and he should be evaluated by an ophthalmologist.

   TREATMENT: You start treatment with NSAIDs as needed and see him back in 2-3 weeks to note any improvement. If he continues to have pain and swelling after 3 months, you may consider adding a longer-term medication like a DMARD.

# 5

# *Systemic Lupus Erythematosus (SLE)*

*Systemic Lupus Erythematous (SLE)* is an autoimmune disease with a wide range of clinical presentations. It affects 0.1-0.25% of the population, depending on the area of the globe and gender/ethnicity. SLE can involve nearly any organ system. Thus, SLE is brought up in the differential of a long list of symptoms. This is especially true if a young African-American female presents with multiple complaints, since SLE is more common in this population; but importantly, SLE can involve any ethnicity at any age.

The pathophysiology of SLE is incompletely understood but thought to be an immune complex-mediated disease. An immune complex is an antibody bound with its antigen. The immune complexes then deposit into tissue, which triggers the immune system to respond with inflammation (increase in macrophages, neutrophils, and lymphocytes) and complement deposition in the area of immune complex deposition. The inflammatory cells target the tissue where the immune complexes have deposited, and damage occurs. (There is a decrease in serum C3 and C4 since these complement components are being used up in the inflammatory process.) It is unclear why immune complexes deposit in certain tissues and not others.

This is an oversimplification of the disease process as some patients with SLE have no histological evidence of immune complex deposition within tissue. All patients with lupus have a positive anti-nuclear antibody (ANA), but it doesn't appear that the ANA is causative in the pathophysiology of SLE.

Importantly, SLE can be diagnosed with just one system involvement (e.g. cutaneous SLE; lupus nephritis) and the appropriate autoimmune serologies (discussed later). More commonly, however, SLE presents with multiple system involvement, such as inflammatory arthritis; rash; low red blood cell, white blood cell and/or platelets counts; as well as lupus nephritis.

## History and Physical Exam in SLE

SLE is a difficult disease to review, since its manifestations vary. The simplest way to discuss the disease is with a systems approach, considering how SLE can involve each system individually. When you are concerned about a patient possibly having SLE, it helps to break it down by the system SLE could be affecting and ask the patient questions, going down the list of organ systems **(Fig. 5-1)**.

*Overall.* SLE more commonly affects young African-American females. Your suspicion should be raised for the possible diagnosis of SLE if an African-American female of childbearing age presents with multiple complaints or unexplained laboratory Abnormalities. SLE can also effect middle aged Caucasian patients, but it's less likely.

*Joints.* Inflammatory arthritis can be one of the dominating symptoms in SLE. There isn't a classic presentation for SLE like we see in other diseases, such as rheumatoid arthritis. SLE can present with either a symmetric polyarticular inflammatory arthritis or an asymmetric oligoarticular inflammatory arthritis.

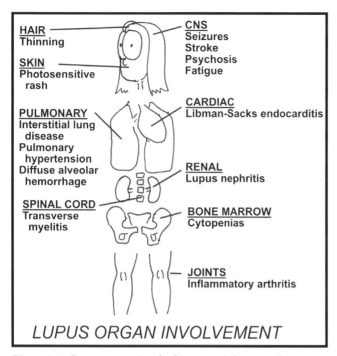

Figure-5-1 Organ systems involved in systemic lupus erythematosus.

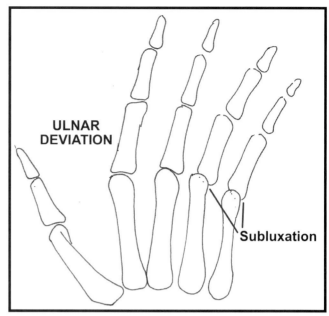

Figure 5-2 Skeletal image of subluxation of the metacarpophalangeal joints in the 4th and 5th digit in SLE.

The joint pain in SLE can be an additive pattern, but it can also be a migratory pattern. In other words, the pattern of joint involvement isn't very helpful in diagnosing SLE; you need other organ involvement to narrow down the diagnosis.

SLE is generally not considered an erosive arthritis, meaning the inflammation in the joint does not erode the bone and cartilage with resultant permanent joint loss as seen in rheumatoid arthritis and spondyloarthritis. Joint abnormalities in SLE can ensue, but this is usually secondary to loosening of the ligaments around the finger joints, which can lead to finger joint subluxation. *Subluxation* is an incomplete dislocation of the joint bones; it occurs in SLE because of laxity of the ligaments around the joint. It is easy to distinguish subluxation versus erosion on plain radiographs. With subluxation, the contours of the bones are normal and not eaten away, which is what occurs in rheumatoid arthritis. With subluxation, plain radiographs show that the metacarpal phalangeal bones appear to overlap one another, like one fell behind the other **(Fig. 5-2)**.

*Jaccoud arthropathy* in SLE refers to reversible ulnar deviation of the metacarpal phalangeal joints of the hands. The examiner, on grasping the patient's fingers, can move the ulnar deviated fingers back into a straight position. In contrast, the ulnar deviation is not reversible in rheumatoid arthritis. Jaccoud arthropathy is reversible because the joints themselves are not damaged; the bones of the joint are subluxed and can be temporarily moved back into place **(Fig. 5-3)**.

*Hematologic abnormalities.* SLE is associated with a wide range of hematologic abnormalities, most notably cytopenias, which are low numbers of white blood cells (*leukopenia*), red blood cells (*anemia*), and/or platelets (*thrombocytopenia*). There are probably multiple mechanisms by which SLE patients develop cytopenias, but the major cause is destruction of the cells by the immune cells (macrophages and neutrophils).

Thrombocytopenia is especially important in SLE, since *Immune Thrombocytopenic Purpura* (an autoimmune destruction of platelets) can precede SLE. In this instance, the patient will be noted to have a low platelet count months to years prior to the diagnosis of SLE.

*Skin.* The classic presentation of lupus is a *malar rash* on the face, also called a *butterfly rash*. The rash is erythematous, usually worsening with sun exposure, and doesn't cross the nasolabial folds of the face **(Fig. 5-4)**. The duration of the facial rash is important to note, since many people with facial flushing may worry that they have the butterfly rash of lupus. Facial flushing usually lasts minutes to hours, whereas the rash from lupus lasts days to weeks.

While the malar rash of lupus is usually mentioned on test questions, lupus can cause a variety of skin rashes anywhere on the body, and there isn't a type of rash you can say with certainty is or isn't lupus, without a biopsy.

Another feature of lupus is *hair loss*. Hair loss can occur in patches around the head, but more commonly the patient will develop thinning of the hair at the hairline on the forehead.

*Renal.* Lupus nephritis is an important cause of morbidity and mortality in patients with SLE. Most

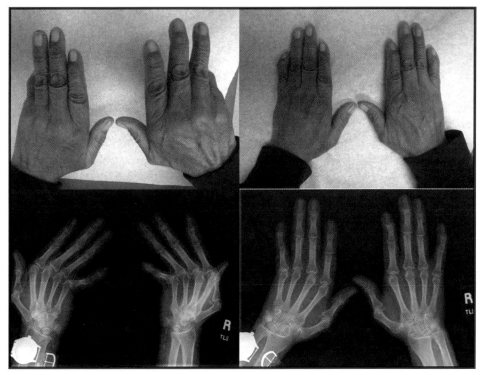

*Figure 5-3 Jaccoud arthropathy. Notice the ulnar deviation, which resolves when the hands are pushed flat against a surface. Image courtesy of the American College of Rheumatology.*

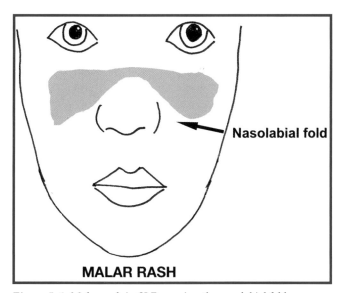

*Figure 5-4 Malar rash in SLE, sparing the nasolabial fold.*

patients with SLE have some renal involvement, but the severity varies greatly from patient to patient. Renal involvement is often asymptomatic, so patients with SLE need to be screened by performing a urinalysis to evaluate for proteinuria. Proteinuria is one of the first signs of lupus involvement in the kidney. If proteinuria is detected, a quantitative study such as a 24-hour urine collection to evaluate the protein level or a random

urine protein/creatinine ratio should be done. Normal urine protein excretion is less than 100 mg/day. Anything above 100 mg/day is considered abnormal and may indicate lupus involvement in the kidney. If the proteinuria is severe enough, a renal biopsy is recommended.

On *biopsy*, histologic findings consistent with the diagnosis of SLE are termed *full house*. Full house refers to the immunofluorescence pattern. Immunofluorescence is a tissue staining technique to see if certain antibodies and protein are deposited and light up (*immunofluorescence*). When examining renal pathology, three antibodies are evaluated (IgG, IgM, IgA) as well as two components of the complement cascade (C1q and C3). In a full house pattern, all of the antibodies and complement components will be positive via immunofluorescence. This contrasts with other autoimmune disease such as ANCA (Anti-Neutrophil Cytoplasmic Antibodies)-associated vasculitis, which will have little, if any, antibody or complement deposition in the kidneys (*pauci-immune*).

*Pulmonary.* One of the most common pulmonary involvements in patients with SLE is pleurisy (*pleuritis*), which is inflammation of the membranes surrounding the lung. Patients with pleuritis complain of sharp pain in the chest that worsens with breathing. This is an important question to ask a patient suspected of having SLE.

As with other autoimmune conditions, patients with SLE can develop inflammation of the lung parenchyma (*interstitial lung disease*), elevations in the pressure of the pulmonary artery (*pulmonary hypertension*), or bleeding within the lung (*diffuse alveolar hemorrhage*).

A unique but rare pulmonary complication of SLE is *shrinking lung syndrome*. A patient with SLE and shrinking lung syndrome will develop shortness of breath, and chest radiographs will show an elevated diaphragm, which can indicate shrinking of the lung space. The pathophysiology of shrinking lung syndrome is unclear but most patients have good outcomes.

Considering the multiple ways the lungs can be involved in SLE, patients with SLE should have at least one chest x-ray and one pulmonary function test to evaluate for pulmonary abnormalities, whether they have symptoms of shortness of breath or not.

*Cardiac.* The important cardiac manifestation of SLE is *Libman-Sacks endocarditis,* a term used to describe sterile vegetations that occur on the mitral valve (usually) of patients with SLE (in contrast to infectious endocarditis, which has vegetations composed of an infectious organism). Usually, these vegetations are asymptomatic, but they can occasionally be associated with embolism and stroke.

*Central Nervous System.* Central nervous system involvement due to SLE can be difficult to prove and should only be diagnosed after other causes of central nervous system pathology are ruled out, such as malignancy, infectious or metabolic causes. CNS involvement in SLE can cause changes in mental status that resemble depression, psychosis, or dementia. No test is available to prove that SLE is causing the mood disorders. To help make the diagnosis, the provider and patient may notice that the patient's mood improves when on more aggressive immunosuppression.

SLE has been implicated in a wide array of CNS manifestations, but SLE involvement of the CNS is a diagnosis of exclusion, since we do not have a test to prove that CNS involvement is due to SLE. Patients need to be worked up for malignancy, infections, or metabolic disorders that could be causing their CNS manifestations before implicating SLE.

*Spinal cord.* Spinal cord involvement in SLE is a rare but potentially devastating complication. SLE can be associated with *transverse myelitis* (inflammatory demyelinating disease of the spine), which may cause the patient to suddenly lose bowel and bladder control along with rapidly progressive weakness of the extremities. These patients need to be evaluated promptly with an MRI of the spine and aggressive glucocorticoid treatment.

Most patients with SLE will not develop many of these complications. More commonly, a patient with SLE will have a photosensitive rash, inflammatory joint pain, pleuritis, mild cytopenias, and possible kidney involvement.

## Laboratory Diagnosis of SLE

*"Doctor, I was told I have lupus because my ANA is positive."* Anti-nuclear antibody (ANA) is an important test in the diagnosis of SLE, not because it means the patient has SLE, but because if it is negative, it means the patient does *not* have SLE. The ANA is a non-specific test that is positive in around 10-20% of the healthy population. The test is, however, very sensitive; if negative, you can say with 99% certainty that the patient does not have SLE.

If the ANA is positive and the patient has a clinical suspicion of SLE, the next test to order is the extractable nuclear antigen (ENA) panel, which is a set of labs that usually includes:

- Anti-SSA/SSB antibody
- Anti-Chromatin antibody
- Anti-Ribonucleoprotein (RNP) antibody
- Anti-Smith antibody (most specific antibody in the ENA panel)

Multiple serologies can be associated with SLE. To simplify, if one of the above ENA panel tests comes back positive, this (in combination with a positive ANA) increases the likelihood that the patient has SLE. Remember the ENA panel as another group of tests that can help point to the diagnosis of SLE. Just to make things more complicated, some of the tests in the ENA can also be associated with other diseases; e.g. SSA/SSB in Sjögren's syndrome. Of all the antibodies in the ENA panel, Anti-Smith is the most specific test for SLE.

*Double-Stranded DNA* is not within the ENA panel but is one of the more specific tests for SLE. A positive Double-Stranded DNA antibody suggests a high likelihood of having SLE; it also predicts renal involvement (proteinuria and possible renal failure).

Note that the diagnosis of SLE is not made solely by lab tests. Clinical suspicion of SLE should be raised when a patient presents with any of the following:

- Photosensitive rash, especially on the face, that lasts for multiple days after exposure to the sun
- Unexplained anemia or thrombocytopenia
- Inflammatory arthritis that may be oligo- or polyarticular and may be migratory
- Progressive unexplained kidney disease with high amounts of protein in the urine
- History of pulmonary embolism or deep vein thrombosis
- New onset of interstitial lung disease or diffuse alveolar hemorrhage

## Following a Patient with SLE

SLE is a chronic disease with a wide range of severity. Some patients will have a mild photosensitive rash and mild thrombocytopenia when exposed to sunlight. At the other extreme, a patient can present with diffuse alveolar hemorrhage and renal failure. Once diagnosed with SLE, the patient needs to be followed every few months and monitored closely. Depending on the severity of the SLE, the patient may require long-term medication to put the disease in remission, but despite the doctor's best efforts the disease can flare. Monitoring a patient's labs can help detect a lupus flare. The following labs give a clue to disease activity:

- *Double-Stranded-DNA antibody* (if the patient has it) can increase in titer when the disease is active. Be sure to check the lab when the patient is thought to be in remission, so you know the baseline number. Then if symptoms worsen and the double-stranded DNA levels increase, this is more evidence for a disease flare.
- *C3 and C4 levels* will decrease when the disease is active. C3 and C4 are part of the complement system and C3 and C4 numbers will decrease when the complement system is being activated (which occurs in active SLE), because components of the complement system are being deposited in tissues such as the kidney.
- *Urinalysis* and *urine protein/creatinine ratio*. A urinalysis should be performed every few months. If proteinuria is detected, the patient should be evaluated by nephrology and considered for a renal biopsy.

# Differential Diagnosis of SLE

## Drug-induced Lupus

A patient may present with cytopenias, inflammatory arthritis, as well as a positive ANA and positive anti-RNP antibody, appearing just like SLE; however, the patient was started on the blood pressure medication hydralazine a few weeks before. This clinical scenario would most likely be a *drug-induced SLE*. Drug-induced SLE can look just like regular SLE, but the patient may be a middle-aged Caucasian male, which isn't the typical SLE demographic—a big clue. The drugs most often implicated are *hydralazine* (a blood pressure medication), *minocycline* (an antibiotic), and *procainamide* (a cardiac medication).

In drug-induced SLE, the patient is less likely to have double-stranded DNA positivity, and more likely to have *anti-histone antibody* (although this is positive in half of idiopathic lupus patients as well). If the anti-histone is negative, then it's unlikely to be drug-induced SLE.

Drug-induced SLE is an important diagnosis to make, since the disease may dissipate with cessation of the drug and the patient may not require long-term immunosuppressive medications. Remember, whenever you have a new diagnosis of SLE, look at the patient's medication list to see if it includes any of the common culprits.

## Antiphospholipid Syndrome

*Antiphospholipid syndrome* is an autoimmune clotting disorder that is associated with antibodies against three phospholipid antigens. The mechanism for the abnormal clot formation is unknown but is likely related to the specific antibody's interaction with phospholipids, which make up the lipid bilayers of cells. How this results in clot formation is unclear. Antiphospholipid syndrome is one of the leading causes of blood clot formation in patients under the age of 50. Patients with this syndrome can have either venous or arterial thrombosis.

Antiphospholipid syndrome is associated with SLE because some of the first patients described with antiphospholipid syndrome also had SLE. SLE patients do have an increased risk of developing the antibodies against phospholipids, but most patients with antiphospholipid syndrome do not have SLE. To add to the confusion, one of the antibodies of antiphospholipid antibody syndrome is called *lupus anticoagulant*, but, again, patients with lupus anticoagulant do not necessarily have lupus. Another confusing aspect of the naming is that it's called *lupus anti-coagulant*, which sounds like the patient would be more prone to bleeding but they do the opposite; they clot! Lupus anti-coagulant is termed *anti-coagulant* because of its function in the laboratory where it extends bleeding time, but in the body it's actually a pro-coagulant. Every aspect of the term *lupus anti-coagulant* is confusing. The two other antibodies associated with phospholipid binding are anti-beta-2 glycoprotein and anti-cardiolipin.

Recurrent miscarriage is another important clinical manifestation of antiphospholipid antibody syndrome. It is important to recognize this because treatment with anticoagulation can increase the chances of a patient having a full-term pregnancy.

Patients tested for antiphospholipid antibody syndrome will be tested for all three of the antibodies. However, to make the diagnosis, only one of these antibodies needs to be present in a high titer in the appropriate clinical scenario (unexplained thrombotic event or miscarriage). To be considered positive, the antibody still has to be present when the test is repeated 12 weeks later.

### Lupus Overlap Syndromes

Autoimmune diseases in general are rare, but patients with one autoimmune disease are at higher risk than the general public for developing another autoimmune disease. A patient with myositis, for instance, can develop scleroderma. Considering that most autoimmune diseases can overlap with any other autoimmune diseases, there isn't a specific term used for the vast majority of overlap syndromes, with the exception of *mixed connective tissue disease*.

The term *mixed connective tissue disease* is confusing because it is not just a mixture of any autoimmune disease with another. It is its own disease entity, overlapping specific autoimmune diseases:

- *Systemic lupus erythematosus*: joint pain, fevers, photosensitive rash
- *Scleroderma*: thickening and hardening of the skin on the hands, Raynaud's
- *Polymyositis*: proximal muscle weakness from muscle inflammation and muscle destruction

The patient with mixed connective tissue disease will develop the above symptoms of the three different autoimmune diseases and will have a positive RNP antibody. Of note, patients with just SLE often have a positive RNP, so to diagnose the patient with mixed connective tissue disease, the patient will need to develop evidence of scleroderma, SLE, and polymyositis (see Chapter 12, Scleroderma; Chapter 14, Inflammatory Myopathies).

# Treatment of SLE

The treatment of SLE depends on the extent of disease and organ involvement.

*General guidelines for patients with SLE:*

- **Sun protection.** Avoidance of direct sunlight is important in SLE. Direct exposure to sunlight can exacerbate the disease.
- **Diet/exercise.** Patients with SLE can be intermittently on glucocorticoids, which contribute to weight gain and muscle atrophy. It is important that patients live a reasonably active, healthy lifestyle to reduce the risks of obesity and muscle loss.

*Non-organ threatening disease.* An example of non-organ threatening disease is a patient with occasional malar rash and joint pains that mostly resolve with use of Non-Steroidal Anti-Inflammatory (NSAID) medications.

**Hydroxychloroquine (Plaquenil).**
Hydroxychloroquine is the backbone of treatment for all patients with SLE. The goal of hydroxychloroquine therapy is to quiet down mild disease, but also reduce the risk of disease progression.

If symptoms are more severe (e.g. the joint pain is severe enough to limit activities of daily living), then more aggressive therapies should be pursued in combination with hydroxychloroquine.

**Methotrexate or Azathioprine.** Methotrexate and azathioprine are more potent medications and are used in patients with more advanced disease, including organ-threatening disease.

**Belimumab** can be used in patients with joint and skin involvement that doesn't respond to hydroxychloroquine monotherapy.

*Organ-threatening disease* encompasses the kidneys, lungs, peripheral and central nervous system. More aggressive management is needed when treating organ-threatening disease.

**High-dose intravenous glucocorticoids.** If organ-threatening disease is detected, the only medication that will provide rapid relief of inflammation and organ damage is glucocorticoids. Intravenous methylprednisolone is a commonly prescribed high dose glucocorticoid that can be given in the hospital to hopefully halt rapid progression of disease.

**Cyclophosphamide.** This is a potent medication used to treat advanced lupus nephritis. It has multiple side effects (see Chapter 2).

**Mycophenolate mofetil (Cellcept)** has been shown to be as effective as cyclophosphamide in the treatment of lupus nephritis with fewer side effects. Mycophenolate mofetil is usually the preferred agent when treating lupus nephritis.

# Cases

1. HISTORY: A 24-year-old African American woman presents with a 3-month history of a facial rash that worsens with sun exposure, as well as mild joint pains in her MCPs that are worse in the morning and better as the day progresses. She reports no recent illnesses and is on no medications.

   LAB: Urinalysis is normal. Her laboratory evaluation shows a positive ANA and a positive anti-chromatin and anti-Smith antibody. Her double-stranded DNA antibody is negative. C3 and C4 are mildly low.

   DIAGNOSIS: This young woman's presentation is consistent with mild SLE. She has a mild inflammatory arthritis, malar rash, and positive lupus serologies. She is double-stranded DNA negative, which makes her less likely to develop renal complications of SLE.

TREATMENT: It is important to initiate treatment with immunosuppressive medications at this point because this may lessen the risk of the disease progressing and developing more organ involvement. *Hydroxychloroquine* (Plaquenil) is a reasonable medication for this patient with mild disease. It is not a potent medication but has few side effects. A low dose of prednisone can be used for a few weeks to calm down the inflammation of her rash and joint pains while the hydroxychloroquine slowly begins to work.

2. HISTORY: A 32-year-old woman with a history of lupus (skin and join involvement, positive ANA and double-stranded DNA), previously on hydroxychloroquine and low dose prednisone, presents to the emergency room with worsening lower extremity edema and shortness of breath.

LAB: Creatinine is 4.5 mg/dl and the urine shows 3+ protein on dip. She is found to have diffuse lower extremity edema and evidence of pulmonary edema on chest x-ray. Cardiac echocardiogram shows a normal ejection fraction. Her double-stranded DNA level is higher than her baseline, and her C3 and C4 are lower than usual. She undergoes renal biopsy, which shows evidence of inflammation from lupus nephritis.

DIAGNOSIS: The patient is presenting with renal failure in the setting of lupus nephritis, which is causing protein loss in her urine and subsequent volume overload, resulting in lower extremity swelling and pulmonary edema.

TREATMENT: She should be treated aggressively with high dose glucocorticoids (intravenous solumedrol 1,000 mg x 3 days), then prednisone 60 mg a day with taper. She should also be started on a long-term aggressive immunosuppressant medication such as *mycophenolate mofetil* (Cellcept) or *cyclophosphamide* (Cytoxan). Mycophenolate mofetil has been shown to be as effective as cyclophosphamide with fewer side effects, which is why it is usually the preferred medication for lupus nephritis.

3. HISTORY: A 54-year-old man with a history of elevated blood pressure presents with pain and swelling in his MCPs that is worse in the morning and better as the day progresses. He has no other symptoms. The patient is taking hydralazine for his blood pressure.

LAB: Hemoglobin and platelet count are low. Autoimmune serologies show elevated ANA as well as anti-chromatin, anti-RNP, and anti-histone.

DIAGNOSIS: This patient's presentation is most consistent with drug-induced SLE secondary to hydralazine. First, discontinue the hydralazine. This will not likely stop the swelling immediately, and he will most likely require prednisone or NSAID therapy to help with the swelling and pain. Hopefully, his symptoms will resolve over the next few weeks to months, but in a minority of patients the drug-induced SLE may persist despite stopping therapy, requiring long-term immunosuppression.

# 6

# *Crystalline Arthritis*

*Crystalline arthritis* differs from previously discussed systemic autoimmune inflammatory arthritides. Crystalline arthritis occurs when crystals form within a joint, triggering an immune response to the crystals, recruiting inflammatory cells to the area, with subsequent pain, warmth, and swelling of the affected joint. Thus, crystal arthritis is caused by an immune response to a foreign material within the joint, in contrast to autoimmune inflammatory arthritides like rheumatoid arthritis, where the immune system is targeting its own tissue.

Crystalline arthritis is unique among rheumatologic conditions because the majority of disease flares are *self-limiting*, i.e. the severe pain and swelling will resolve without any treatment and the joint will return to normal. This is a big clue to the diagnosis. If a patient presents with severe monoarticular joint pain that lasted 4 days, completely resolving after a few more days, crystalline disease should be high on your differential. The two most common crystalline diseases are gout and pseudogout, which will be discussed separately. Crystalline disease can involve any joint in the body (but gout has an affinity for the big toe and pseudogout has an affinity for the knees), and usually presents monoarticular or asymmetric oligoarticular **(Fig. 6-1)**.

## Gout

Gout is the most common form of inflammatory arthritis, occurring in about 5% of the general population. The incidence increases greatly with age.

Gout is caused by the deposition of monosodium urate crystals in joints, with a subsequent immune response to the crystals. The inflammatory reaction to gout is severe and disabling and is considered the most painful condition in rheumatology.

Gout is most common in men but can occur in women, usually after menopause (estrogen increases renal secretion of uric acid). As people age, their risk of gout increases, likely because of aging kidneys and decreased ability of the kidney to excrete uric acid, thus increasing serum uric acid levels.

*Diet and Gout.* Prior to the development of medications to treat gout, it was known that avoidance of certain foods decreases the occurrence of gout flares. Diets that consist of high levels of meat, beer, and seafood are associated with higher levels of serum uric acid and greater risks of gout flares. Dairy products, in contrast, are associated with lower serum uric acid levels. Unfortunately, in most patients, dietary restriction isn't enough to control serum uric acid levels, and the patient will need a medication to lower the serum uric acid.

## Pathophysiology of Gout

When serum uric acid levels rise beyond their solubility in serum (6.8 mg/dL), the serum urate precipitates as monosodium urate crystals. This doesn't always occur though. You will see many patients with elevated uric acid levels well above 6.8 mg/dL without any clinical evidence of gout. The monosodium urate precipitates in the joint; the immune system recognizes

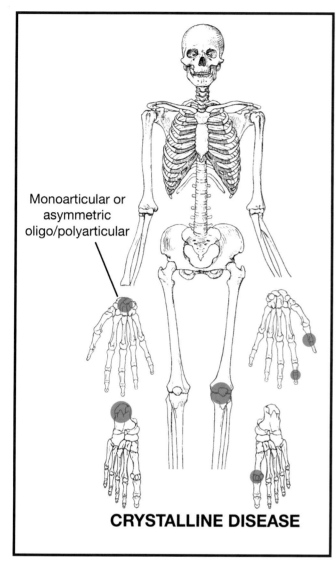

Monoarticular or
asymmetric
oligo/polyarticular

**CRYSTALLINE DISEASE**

*Figure 6-1. Crystalline disease is commonly monoarticular, but when multiple joints are involved it is often asymmetric oligo/polyarticular.*

the crystals as foreign and mounts an immune response to the crystals. The immune response consists of multiple inflammatory cells going into the joint causing swelling, redness and severe pain.

## History in Gout

Gout presents in the following characteristic ways:

- Most commonly, the first time a patient experiences a gout attack involves a sudden monoarticular swelling, warmth, and severe pain.
- Classically, the first metatarsal phalangeal (MTP) joint is targeted (*podagra*).
- Without treatment, a gout flare can last up to 2 weeks.

- After the first flare, most patients will have another flare within a year.
- The disease can progress to becoming oligo-polyarticular with subsequent flares.

*Tophi.* When patients have had multiple gout flares over the course of many years, monosodium urate crystals can progressively deposit, causing the formation of a palpable, usually painless nodule near a joint (for example, immediately next to the elbow, but not within the joint). Another area where tophi are often found is the ear lobes, which can be palpated on exam; patients often don't notice the small nodule in the ear lobe.

## Laboratory in Gout

*Serum uric acid.* Gout flares correlate with serum uric acid levels, which fluctuate depending on diet and the amount of cell turnout of uric acid. (Chemotherapy, for instance, increases the number of cells that are dying and releasing intracellular uric acid.) Serum uric acid, however, cannot be used to diagnose gout or a gout flare. In patients with a gout flare, the serum uric acid may be high, normal, or low, so it is not a dependable test for the diagnosis. Serum uric acid levels are useful for monitoring treatment of gout when a patient is on urate-lowering therapies (see below).

*Polarized microscopy* is critical in evaluating a patient with suspected crystalline arthritis. When a patient presents with acute swelling and pain in a single joint, fluid can be drained from the joint (arthrocentesis). Then a sample of synovial fluid is placed under a microscope and illuminated with polarized light that is traveling in a known direction across the sample (the direction is labeled on the microscope). Crystals within the synovial fluid will reflect light differently depending on their composition and can be categorized as either *positively* or *negatively birefringent*.

The observer knows if a crystal is positively or negatively birefringent by the orientation of the crystal to the polarized light (lying parallel or perpendicular), and if the crystal is yellow or blue. If the crystal lies parallel to the direction of the light source and the crystal is blue, then the crystal is positively birefringent. If the crystal is yellow when lying parallel to the light direction, then it is labeled negatively birefringent **(Fig. 6-2)**. If the crystals orient themselves 90 degrees away from the direction they were facing earlier (the crystals are floating in synovial fluid, so they are freely moving), they will turn from yellow to blue, or blue to yellow **(Fig. 6-3)**.

When the crystals move in the fluid and change color, their birefringence stays the same because birefringence

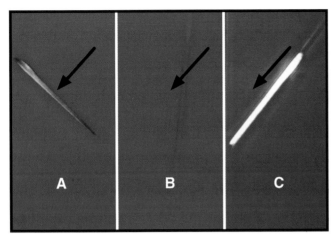

*Figure 6-2. Polarized microscopy with crystal in different positions. Arrows indicate direction of light. When a negatively birefringent crystal is aligned with the light (C) it will be yellow. When perpendicular to the light (A), it will be blue. When in-between (B) it will be hard to see. Image courtesy of the American College of Rheumatology.*

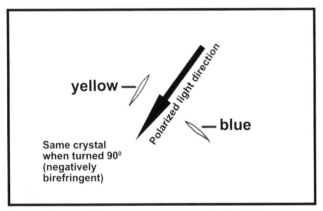

*Figure 6-3. The crystal in relation to the polarized light.*

is determined by the orientation of the polarized light, so a negatively birefringent crystal is always a negatively birefringent crystal. In addition to birefringence, the shape of the crystal helps to make the diagnosis. Gout crystals are needle-shaped; pseudogout crystals are rhomboid **(Fig. 6-4)**.

**X-rays** are useful in patients with gout, especially in the setting of multiple gout attacks over months to years. In the acute setting, the x-ray will only show soft tissue swelling around the joint. In patients suffering from gout attacks for months to years, however, characteristic erosions can be seen around the joints. Erosions are bite-like indentions within the bone. Importantly, in gout the erosions are *near* the joint but *not within* the joint (*peri-articular*). This contrasts with rheumatoid arthritis, where the erosions are *within* the joint (*articular*) **(Fig. 6-5)**.

## Treatment of Gout

The treatment of gout can be divided into two categories, *preventative* and *acute*.

### Preventative Treatment

Serum uric acid levels correspond with the risk of subsequent flares in patients with gout. The goal of *preventative treatment* is to reduce the serum uric acid levels, thus preventing subsequent flares. If the patient's uric acid levels are lowered below 6 mg/dL, then the risk of flares decreases.

Importantly, when a patient starts urate-lowering therapy, there will be a greater risk of flaring within the first few weeks of initiating treatment. Whenever serum uric acid levels drop or rise rapidly, a gout attack can be precipitated. When starting on urate-lowering therapy, the patient should be warned of this risk but also given a rapid-acting medication (*colchicine* or *prednisone*) at the same time to take daily, which will limit the chances of a flare.

Another important aspect of management is to continue the urate-lowering therapy during a flare. Many patients feel compelled to stop the urate-lowering therapy during a gout flare, but if the medication is started and stopped and then restarted, it will just precipitate more flares.

*Serum uric acid* should be followed every few months in patients with gout to evaluate if urate-lowering therapy is effective.

All patients should be educated about potential gout triggers in their diets, such as red meat, seafood, and alcohol. Diet alone will likely not completely control the disease, and the patient will require urate-lowering medications **(Fig. 6-6)**.

### Acute Treatment

Acute treatment can be used in the acute setting of a gout flare to decrease the severity and longevity of a flare **(Fig. 6-7)**.

| FIGURE 6-4. GOUT VS PSEUDOGOUT: POLARIZED MICROSCOPY | |
|---|---|
| **Crystal Disease** | **Features under the microscope** |
| Gout | Negatively birefringent (yellow parallel with polarized light), needle-shaped |
| Pseudogout (CPPD) | Positively birefringent (blue parallel with polarized light), rhomboid-shaped |

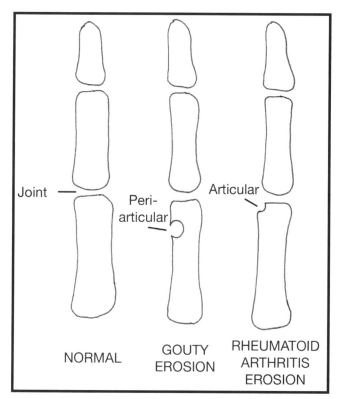

*Figure 6-5. Gouty erosion. The erosion is near the joint (periarticular), in comparison to an erosion from rheumatoid arthritis, which is within the joint (articular).*

# Pseudogout (CPPD)

*Calcium pyrophosphate dehydrate (CPPD)* or *pseudogout* is a crystalline disease that is common in the elderly

and is likely under-recognized. CPPD can behave like gout; it can cause an acute debilitating self-limiting monoarticular or polyarticular inflammatory arthritis, but it can also present as a chronic inflammatory arthritis that may resemble rheumatoid arthritis. In fact, this disease is the rheumatologic version of tuberculosis; it seems to be able to mimic a variety of diseases, as we will discuss.

## *Pathophysiology of Pseudogout*

The pathophysiology of pseudogout is more complex and incompletely understood compared to gout. Currently it's thought that the joint cartilage produces excess pyrophosphate that crystalizes, which elicits an immune response similar to monosodium urate crystal deposition. It's unclear what triggers the joint cartilage to make excess pyrophosphate, but it's known to be associated with other conditions, such as low serum magnesium, hyperparathyroidism, hypophosphatasia, hemochromatosis, and previous trauma to a joint.

## *History in Pseudogout*

*Pseudogout (CPPD)* can present as an acute monoarticular self-limiting inflammatory arthritis that rapidly worsens over the course of hours, appearing identical to gout. The pain and swelling may last for 1-2 weeks and then subside on its own. CPPD involves the knee more than the metatarsophalangeal (MTP) joint of the great toe, seen in gout. The only way to differentiate

| FIGURE 6-6. LONG-TERM URATE LOWERING MEDICATIONS | |
|---|---|
| **Drug Name** | **Mechanism of Urate Lowering** |
| Allopurinol and febuxostat | Inhibit xanthine oxidase (Allopurinol use is limited in patients with kidney disease as the drug is cleared through the kidneys; febuxostat can be used in patients with kidney disease.) |
| Probenecid | Increases renal secretion of uric acid |
| Pegloticase | Converts uric acid to the soluble allantoin, which is readily excreted in the urine. This drug is given as an infusion and is reserved for severe cases. |
| Lesinurad | Inhibitor of URAT1 and OAT4 uric acid transporters of the kidney; increases renal excretion of uric acid |

| FIGURE. 6-7 TREATMENT OPTIONS FOR GOUT FLARES | |
|---|---|
| **Drug Name** | **Mechanism of Action** |
| Non-steroidal anti-inflammatory drugs (NSAIDs) | Prevent recruitment of inflammatory cells in response to the crystals (cannot be used in kidney disease) |
| Colchicine | Inhibits neutrophil migration into the joint and decreases inflammation (cannot be used in patients with kidney disease) |
| Glucocorticoids | Can be given orally or injected into the joint; can be given in patients with kidney disease |
| Anakinra (interleukin-1 inhibitor) | Interleukin-1 is critical to the inflammatory response that occurs in gout. Blocking IL-1 can rapidly decrease the pain and swelling in an acute attack. |

conclusively is with arthrocentesis and visualization of CPPD crystals on polarized microscopy.

As the name of the disease suggests, CPPD is caused by deposition of the *crystal calcium pyrophosphate dehydrate*. This crystal differs from urate crystals in appearance under the microscope and how it forms. Unlike uric acid, diet doesn't seem to affect the amount of CPPD deposition, and we don't have a serum test that we can follow in patients with CPPD.

## Laboratory in Pseudogout

There is no blood test diagnostic of pseudogout. The diagnosis of pseudogout relies on synovial fluid analysis. Polarized microscopic analysis of CPPD crystals reveals a rhomboid, positively birefringent (blue when parallel with polarized light) crystal. CPPD crystals are more difficult to identify than monosodium urate crystals because they are smaller and are often not as birefringent (brightly reflected under the microscope) as monosodium urate crystals.

**X-rays** can help evaluate a patient suspected of having CPPD. *Chondrocalcinosis* can be seen on most x-rays in patients with CPPD. Chondrocalcinosis is a thin layer of calcification that deposits between certain joints. Chondrocalcinosis doesn't necessarily cause joint pain, but it is often found incidentally on x-rays done for other reasons; it may suggest CPPD crystals being deposited. Chondrocalcinosis is not diagnostic of pseudogout; it just raises suspicion of the diagnosis.

If you have a patient with episodic, self-limiting joint pain and the patient has a normal serum uric acid, and the patient is not in the office when they have a flare so you can't get a synovial fluid sample, then ordering x-rays of the knees and wrists is a reasonable approach in the workup. Of note, the pain does not need to occur in the knees or wrists; it can be in the ankle or fingers, but the knee **(Fig. 6-8)** and wrist **(Fig. 6-9)** have the highest yield of finding chondrocalcinosis, no matter where the disease is bothering the patient.

There is an area on the ulnar side of the wrist called the *triangular fibrocartilage*, where chondrocalcinosis can be seen on x-ray. The triangular fibrocartilage is a small triangle shape on the proximal ulnar aspect of the wrist that doesn't have any bones in it **(Fig. 6-8)**.

## Variations of Pseudogout

### Pseudo-rheumatoid Arthritis

Older patients with pseudogout can present with what sounds like a polyarticular symmetric inflammatory arthritis, e.g. rheumatoid arthritis. They complain of morning stiffness, pain in the metacarpal

phalangeal (MCPs) joints and wrists symmetrically. Importantly, they will have negative serologies (negative rheumatoid factor and anti-cyclic citrullinated peptide) for rheumatoid arthritis. Radiographs may show chondrocalcinosis of the wrists, and there will be no erosions on the MCPs, as you would expect to see in advanced rheumatoid arthritis. Arthrocentesis of the wrist will show calcium pyrophosphate dehydrate crystals, indicating pseudogout.

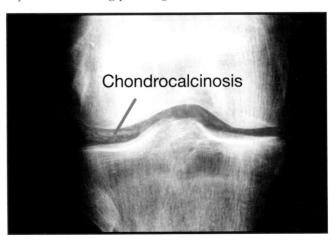

***Figure 6-8.*** *Chondrocalcinosis of the knee. Notice the chalky substance between the femur and the tibia.*

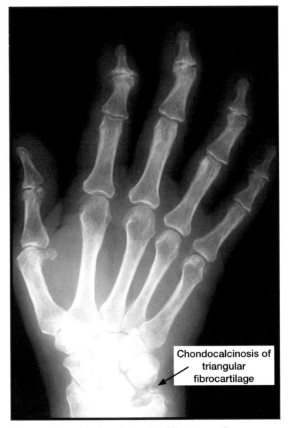

***Figure 6-9.*** *Chondrocalcinosis of the triangular fibrocartilage of the wrist.*

It is important to think about CPPD whenever you see an elderly patient with seronegative rheumatoid arthritis. You might be missing CPPD, which has a completely different treatment strategy. In rheumatoid arthritis, you would expect the pain to be daily, but with pseudogout the patient may describe some days of morning stiffness, swelling, and pain, but then a few days pain-free.

### Osteoarthritis of Pseudogout

Osteoarthritis is the wear and tear arthritis that occurs nearly universally in various joints as people age. For unclear reasons, the metacarpal phalangeal (MCP) joints of the hands are usually spared in osteoarthritis. If you see bony enlargement of the MCPs of an elderly patient that appears like osteoarthritis on physical exam and x-rays, then you should have a high suspicion for CPPD. Another important cause of osteoarthritis of the MCPs is *hemochromatosis*.

### Pseudo-meningitis

CPPD can mimic meningitis when CPPD crystals deposit around the cervical spine in a syndrome called *crowned dens*. An older patient can present with fever and neck stiffness/pain, with an elevated white blood cell count. There may be a diagnostic clue if the patient has a CPPD flare in another joint such as the knee. These patients are understandably initially worked up and treated for meningitis, but their lumbar puncture results are usually unremarkable. The diagnosis can be made by obtaining a CT scan of the neck, which will show the characteristic calcium deposits (*chondrocalcinosis*) around the cervical spine, looking like a crown around the dens of C2, hence the name *crowned dens* (Fig. 6-10).

## *Treatment of Pseudogout (CPPD)*

CPPD is treated in the acute setting similarly to gout, with glucocorticoids or colchicine. There is no

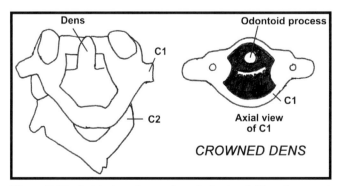

*Figure 6-10. Axial view of normal cervical spine (left) and crowned dens (chondrocalcinosis around the dens) on right.*

preventative medication for CPPD. Some patients with frequent flares may benefit from daily colchicine therapy. Importantly, uric acid-lowering therapy does not help CPPD patients and just places them at risk for side effects of the medication.

## Cases

1. HISTORY: A 64-year-old man with a history of coronary artery disease presents with an acutely swollen and painful big toe. A similar episode occurred about 8 months ago, which improved with ibuprofen.
   LAB: Arthrocentesis is performed in the office, and synovial fluid is examined under the microscope. Negatively birefringent crystals are noted along with a white blood cell count of 14,000 cells/mm$^3$.
   DIAGNOSIS: Gout.
   TREATMENT: In a patient experiencing monoarticular joint pain from gout, steroids (such as *Kenalog*) can be injected into the joint, which will provide rapid relief of the joint pain. Other options would be to give colchicine or oral prednisone. Colchicine is best given at the immediate onset of joint pain. If the joint pain has been ongoing for days, colchicine may take multiple days to start working. Urate-lowering therapy should also be discussed with the patient.

2. HISTORY: A 72-year-old man with a history of crystal-proven gout is hospitalized after recently undergoing cardiac surgery. Before the surgery his allopurinol was stopped, and after the surgery he is started on diuretic medications to help with lower extremity edema. Within 2 days of initiating diuretic therapy, he develops acute onset severe pain in his left ankle. You are called to evaluate the patient. His kidney function has worsened after the surgery.
   LAB: Arthrocentesis of the left ankle reveals negatively birefringent needle-shaped crystals, with a white blood cell count of 12,000/mm$^3$.
   DIAGNOSIS: Gout
   TREATMENT: This is a very common scenario in a hospital. Crystalline disease has a tendency to flare after surgeries, likely because of a combination of fluid shifts that may change serum uric acid levels, but also because of acute kidney injury that decreases renal excretion of uric acid. Even though the patient has a history of gout, his monoarticular joint pain cannot be assumed to be crystalline disease, especially after a major surgery that increases the risk of infection. In order to evaluate the synovial fluid for the white blood cell count

| FIGURE 6-11. PRESENTATIONS OF GOUT, PSEUDOGOUT, INFECTION, AND RA | | | | |
|---|---|---|---|---|
| | **Gout** | **Pseudogout** | **Infection** | **Rheumatoid Arthritis** |
| **Onset** | Abrupt onset, maximum tenderness within 24 hours | Abrupt onset and offset resembling gout, or more insidious with daily pain resembling rheumatoid arthritis | Gradually worsening over days, steady progression without treatment | Insidious onset, usually weeks to months of progressive joint pain, usually daily |
| **Joints involved** | Usually starts with 1 joint (1$^{st}$ MTP is classic) | Most commonly involved joint is the knee, but can involve multiple joints | Almost always just 1 joint | Multiple MCPs involved |
| **Duration** | Pain and swelling lasts 4 days to 2 weeks, then resolves | Lasts 4 days to 2 weeks like gout; can also develop into a daily pain similar to rheumatoid arthritis | Pain and swelling continues to worsen without treatment | Daily persistent pain and swelling, improves with activity |
| **X-ray** | Punched out erosions that are *periarticular and not within the joint* | Chondrocalcinosis (calcium deposition within joints, especially the knees and wrists) | Rapidly progressing joint space loss and erosions | Erosions within the joint, *articular erosions* |
| **Synovial fluid** | WBC 2,000-50,000 cells/mm$^3$ Crystals: negatively birefringent (yellow parallel with polarized light), needle-shaped | WBC 2,000-50,000 cells/mm$^3$ Crystals: positively birefringent (blue parallel with polarized light), rhomboid-shaped | WBC >50,000 cells/mm$^3$ Crystals: none | WBC 2,000-50,000 cells/mm$^3$ Crystals: none |

and presence of crystals, as well as to send the fluid for culture, an arthrocentesis should be performed. If the synovial fluid white blood cell count is less than 50,000 cells/mm$^3$ and crystals are seen, then the risk of a septic joint is much less.

In this post-op patient with an elevated creatinine, joint injection may help. Colchicine and NSAIDs should be avoided in patients with acute kidney injury. Oral glucocorticoids such as prednisone are also a reasonable option, especially in someone with multiple joints involved, as multiple joints would require multiple injections. Prednisone may reduce the body's ability to heal after major surgery, so surgeons are not usually enthusiastic about steroid use after surgery.

3. HISTORY: A 72-year-old man presents with acute left knee swelling and pain for the past 2 days, not improved with ibuprofen. He notes a history of fluctuating pain in his wrists and MCPs. His primary care physician thought he might have rheumatoid arthritis but says his labs for the rheumatoid arthritis were negative.

IMAGING: You look back at the patient's x-rays and note chondrocalcinosis in the wrists. Your suspicion is raised for possible CPPD with subsequent flare of pseudogout in his knee.

LAB: You perform arthrocentesis and note positively birefringent, rhomboid-shaped crystals on synovial fluid analysis. The diagnosis of CPPD is made. The patient's kidney function is normal.

TREATMENT: He can be given colchicine for the acute attack. If his attacks become more frequent, he can take a low dose daily colchicine to prevent attacks. Urate-lowering therapy will have no benefit for this condition.

# 7

# Infectious Causes of Inflammatory Joint Pain

Infection is high on the differential in rheumatology regardless of the presenting symptoms. Infection can mimic many, if not all, diseases in rheumatology and is crucial to recognize, since a diagnosis of infection dramatically changes the treatment. In this chapter, we will discuss infection in the context of joint inflammation.

## Septic Joint

A septic joint is a joint infected with a pathogen that can cause rapid destruction of joint cartilage and synovium. It presents as rapidly worsening pain and swelling in a single joint (monoarticular). The pain is often severe enough that the joint cannot bear weight, with severely limited range of motion.

The most common causes of septic arthritis are *Staphylococcus aureus* and to a lesser degree *Streptococcal* species. Other infectious causes are less common:

- *Gram negative infections* are associated with IV drug use, except for *Neisseria gonorrhoeae,* which is associated with a younger, sexually active population.
- *Fungal infections*. Many types of fungi can cause a septic joint. This usually occurs in immunocompromised patients with a disseminated fungal infection that seeds to the joints.
- *Septic arthritis* or *crystalline disease (gout)* should be highest on the differential of any patient with acute monoarticular inflammatory joint pain.

## Diagnosis of Septic Arthritis

Unfortunately, there is no clinical presentation of a monoarticular inflammatory arthritis that characteristically differentiates septic arthritis from crystalline disease. (Both can have fevers and elevated serum white blood cell counts.) You need to perform an arthrocentesis (drawing fluid out of the joint with a needle) to help differentiate the two conditions.

Synovial fluid immediately helps to differentiate a septic from a non-septic joint. The septic joint usually has a very high white blood cell count (greater than 50,000 wbc/mm$^3$, but can sometimes occur with counts as low as 25,000 wbc/mm$^3$), while autoimmune and crystalline arthritis will have synovial fluid WBC counts between 2,000-50,000 wbc/mm$^3$.

The synovial fluid WBC count therefore overlaps in diagnostic possibilities when it is between 25,000 wbc/mm$^3$ and 50,000 wbc/mm$^3$. Evaluating for crystals in these cases can help differentiate the cause, as can sending the synovial fluid for gram stain and culture. The clinical scenario is also very important: If the patient has had a recent illness such as pneumonia or a skin infection that may have seeded the affected joint, this should raise suspicion for a septic joint. The joint is less likely to be septic if the patient is able to use the joint and bear weight on the joint.

### Treatment of Septic Arthritis

Rapid initiation of antibiotics is critical in the treatment of septic arthritis as well as consultation by orthopedic surgery for surgical evaluation of the joint.

## Infective Endocarditis

*Infective endocarditis* is an infection within a heart valve, usually caused by bacteria. Infective endocarditis often presents with a very sick patient experiencing high fevers and elevated white blood cell count. In a minority of patients, joint pain may be the presenting symptom. The joints may present with generalized aches with no swelling (arthralgias) or with an inflammatory arthritis with swelling, warmth and pain in the joint occurring in an additive or migratory pattern. Joint fluid cultures rarely grow the causal organism. Other clues to the diagnosis on physical exam:

- *Petechiae*: the presence of small red dots on the skin
- *Splinter hemorrhages*: darkened streaks on the nails
- *Osler's nodes*: palpable nodules on the tips of fingers
- *Janeway lesions*: erythematous lesions on the palms and soles that are non-tender

Diagnosis should be suspected in a patient with joint pains, skin changes, high fevers, and a detectable heart murmur. The diagnosis is made with blood cultures and a cardiac echocardiogram that reveals vegetations on the valves.

## Migratory Inflammatory Arthritis

*Migratory inflammatory arthritis* is a rare clinical presentation, usually presenting as a swollen, painful joint lasting for multiple days, followed by resolution of the pain and swelling for hours to days. Then the swelling and pain returns in a *different* joint **(Fig. 7-1)**. Two diagnoses should come to mind: *rheumatic fever* and *gonococcal arthritis*. Other infectious forms of arthritis can present with a migratory pattern, such as infective endocarditis and noninfectious inflammatory arthritis (e.g. ANCA vasculitis and SLE), but these diseases mostly do not present with a migratory pattern; as opposed to rheumatic fever and gonococcal arthritis, both of which are most commonly migratory.

## Gonorrhea

*Gonococcal arthritis* results from the disseminated spread of the sexually transmitted pathogen, *Neisseria gonorrhoeae* **(Fig. 7-2)**. Think about gonococcal arthritis in any young, sexually active patient who presents with

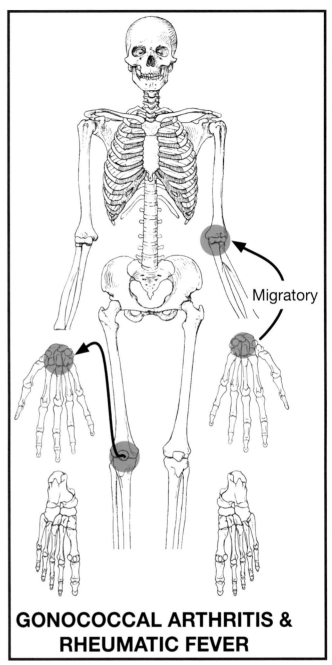

**GONOCOCCAL ARTHRITIS & RHEUMATIC FEVER**

*Figure 7-1.* Migratory arthritis presents with a tender, swollen joint that lasts a few days, resolves, then returns in a different joint.

acute oligo- or polyarticular inflammatory arthritis. In females, the dissemination often occurs around the time of the menstrual period; it's a good question to ask a female patient with new onset inflammatory joint pain if she had her period within the last 7 days.

- Patients with disseminated gonococcus usually appear very sick and have generalized symptoms such as fevers, chills, and malaise.
- Physical exam may reveal an oligo- or polyarticular asymmetric arthritis (one wrist will be involved but

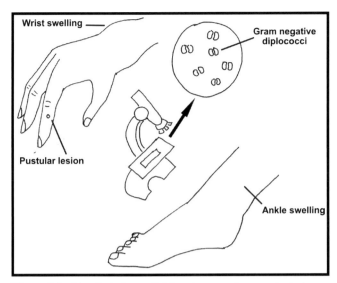

*Figure 7-2. Manifestations of Neisseria gonorrhea may include skin pustules and joint swelling.*

not the other wrist, in contrast with rheumatoid arthritis). Importantly, the patient may have a *tenosynovitis* (inflammation of the tendons, particularly involving the wrists and ankles) that may remit on its own.

- Another diagnostic clue is the skin findings of disseminated gonococcus. The patient may not be aware of a painless, small pustular lesion, usually in the distal extremities.

## Diagnosis and Treatment of Disseminated Gonococcus

It can difficult to prove the diagnosis of disseminated gonococcus; multiple samples from various sites may need to be obtained. The highest yield will come from testing for *Neisseria gonorrhoeae* in a cervical swab (in females) or the urine in males. These sites should be tested even if the patient has no symptoms, such as vaginal or penile discharge. Synovial fluid should be collected via arthrocentesis and sent to the lab for culture and gram staining; the yield in synovial fluid is only around 50%.

Patients should be treated with *ceftriaxone* 1 gram (either intravenously or intramuscularly) every 24 hours along with *azithromycin* 1 gram orally.

## Rheumatic Fever

*Rheumatic fever* differs from the previously mentioned causes of infectious arthritis. The joint pain in rheumatic fever is not caused by an organism itself, but the immune response to a previous infection, namely group A streptococcal pharyngitis. Rheumatic fever occurs in a small proportion of patients with pharyngitis caused by group

A streptococcus (strep throat), when the immune system makes antibodies to group A streptococcus. Some of these antibodies also attack multiple parts of the body, likely because proteins on the bacteria resemble other proteins in the body as in the joints and the heart. This elicits an inflammatory response to the affected area. The incidence of rheumatic fever is decreasing in parts of the world with easy access to antibiotics to treat strep pharyngitis.

## Diagnosis of Rheumatic Fever

The diagnosis of rheumatic fever can be difficult to make, especially considering the incidence of the disease is much lower than in the past, and many physicians are not experienced in recognizing this disease. The diagnosis can be made based on the *Jones criteria*, which has major and minor components, as well as by documentation of previous group A streptococcal infection **(Fig 7-3)**. We will discuss some of the major criteria as well as techniques to demonstrate group A streptococcal infection.

*Joint pain.* The joint pain classically presents 3 weeks after the throat infection. The pain classically involves the medium and large joints, and the pattern is migratory (e.g. left knee pain for 3 days, which resolves, then involves the right elbow). Fluid analysis will often be inflammatory (2,000-50,000 white blood cells/mm$^3$), but no organisms will be grown on the culture. Also, unique to the joint pain in rheumatic fever, the pain will resolve rapidly with salicylate therapy such as aspirin.

*Carditis.* Heart involvement in rheumatic fever carries the highest morbidity and mortality of any of the criteria. Any part of the heart can be involved: the problems range from valvular disease (mitral or aortic regurgitation), myocarditis (decreased overall function of the heart presenting as heart failure), and pericarditis (inflammation of the lining around the heart, causing chest pain).

*Sydenham's chorea is a* neuropsychiatric manifestation of rheumatic fever. It presents as involuntary movements of the extremities and emotional lability. Luckily the symptoms of Syndenham's chorea are often self-limited after 1-3 months.

*Erythema marginatum* is a unique rash to look for when evaluating a patient for possible rheumatic fever. It appears as an erythematous, sharply demarcated, and blanching serpiginous rash. *Serpiginous* refers to snake-like, meaning the rash appears to snake up or down the affected part of the body. Whenever you hear of a rash being serpiginous, you should think of erythema marginatum and rheumatic fever!

*Documenting previous group A streptococcal infection is critical in diagnosing rheumatic fever.*

*Positive throat culture.* Throat culture is obtained by swabbing the back of a patient's mouth and then

## FIGURE 7-3. MODIFIED JONES CRITERIA FOR DIAGNOSING RHEUMATIC FEVER

Must prove previous exposure to Group A strep + 2 Major criteria OR 1 Major criteria + 2 minor criteria

| Major Criteria | Manifestations |
|---|---|
| Polyarthritis | Migratory inflammatory arthritis (swollen, warm, painful joints) |
| Carditis (heart involvement) | Evidence of congestive heart failure (lower extremity swelling, pulmonary edema), or pericarditis, or new valvular abnormality |
| Subcutaneous nodules | Painless nodules present on the back of the wrist, elbows, or knees |
| Erythema marginatum | A "serpentine," erythematous, well demarcated rash that appears to snake up and down a part of the body |
| Syndenham's chorea | Involuntary movement of the face or arms (*chorea* means "to dance") |
| **Minor Criteria** | |
| Fever | Greater than 38.2 degrees Celsius or 100.8 degrees Fahrenheit |
| Arthralgia | Joint pain without swelling and warmth (arthralgias), differing from inflammatory arthritis Arthralgia cannot be used as a minor criterion if polyarthritis is used as a major criterion. |
| Elevated Inflammatory markers | Elevation of either the Erythrocyte Sedimentation Rate of the C-reactive protein |
| Leukocytosis | Elevation of the serum white blood cell count |
| ECG showing evidence of heart block | May feel palpitations |

placing the swab on a culture medium. A throat culture has a higher yield before antibiotics are administered. Remember, the joint pain from rheumatic fever occurs 3-4 weeks after the initial throat infection, so performing the throat culture when the joint pain occurs has a low yield for making the diagnosis (25%).

*Rapid Strep antigen detection tests.* These tests can be done in the physician's office, much more quickly than waiting for a culture, which takes up to 48 hours to return.

*Streptococcal antibody tests.* If the culture and rapid strep tests are inconclusive, testing the patient's serum for antibodies to streptococcus can be helpful. The most commonly used test is the *anti-streptolysin O (ASO)*. The titers of the test will increase with time if a recent infection occurred, which can be very helpful when evaluating for rheumatic fever. If a patient had a sore throat 3 weeks ago, the ASO may be negative; but then testing 2 weeks later the test will be moderately positive; and then retesting another week later will demonstrate a high positive lab number, which supports a recent infection and a subsequent mounting immune response.

# Organisms Causing Slowly Progressive Joint Damage

The following organisms can disseminate through the blood and cause joint infection, but they differ from Staphylococcus, Streptococcus, and N. *gonorrhoeae* in that the infections are not nearly as rapidly progressive. A patient experiencing infections with the following organisms can present with pain and swelling progressing over the course of weeks or months compared to the rapid hours-to-days progression seen with Staph, Strep, or Neisseria gonorrhea.

## Mycobacterium Tuberculosis

The primary osteoarticular site for tuberculosis spread is the spine, but large joints can also be involved, mainly the hips and knees. Small joints like the hands are rarely affected. Patients often do not have concomitant pulmonary symptoms. A normal chest radiograph does not exclude the diagnosis of septic arthritis from mycobacterium tuberculosis.

## Nontuberculosis Mycobacterium

Multiple types of nontuberculous mycobacterium can cause a septic arthritis **(Fig. 7-8)**.

Like mycobacterium tuberculosis, nontuberculous mycobacterium usually manifests as a slowly progressive swelling of the joints. Unlike mycobacterium tuberculosis, nontuberculous mycobacterium is less likely to involve the vertebrae. Nontuberculous mycobacterium has a higher propensity to develop a tenosynovitis (inflammation of the tendon as well as the synovium).

Nontuberculous mycobacterium can cause *nodular lymphangitis*, which consists of several painful nodular lesions along the lymph nodes that drain the site of infection.

Classically, *Mycobacterium marinum* will present after trauma to the skin exposed to salt water or a fish tank. The area of trauma develops painful skin nodules that extend away from the site, and a nearby joint can become swollen and painful.

## Lyme Disease

*Lyme disease* is caused by the spirochete *Borrelia burgdorferi* and is transmitted by the tick *Ixodes scapularis*. The prevalence of the disease depends on its location in the country **(Fig. 7-4)**, with a much higher incidence in the northeastern United States, where Ixodes scapularis is more common.

"Are you sure it's not Lyme disease doctor?"

No matter what your role in the health care field is going to be, it's a good idea to familiarize yourself with Lyme disease, since the clinical presentation can vary. Lyme disease also comes up in internet symptom searches performed by the patient, who will often ask the physician about what he/she finds.

Lyme disease can present in multiple different stages, depending on how long the infection has existed:

- In the *early localized stage* of Lyme disease, patients develop a typical skin lesion called *erythema marginatum*, which looks like a bullseye target, that develops anywhere on the body after inoculation by the tick. Patients may experience fatigue and arthralgias during this time.
- In *early disseminated disease*, cardiac manifestations may arise (conduction abnormalities) as well as neurologic problems (encephalopathy, extremity weakness).
- In *late disease*, persistent arthritis can occur, usually in a large joint, such as the knee.
- The *inflammatory arthritis of Lyme disease* can be severe and can develop either early or late in the

infection. The key to recognizing the inflammatory arthritis is that it is usually monoarticular to oligoarticular, involving the large joints, especially the knee. The arthritis can also be migratory, with inflammation and swelling moving from one large joint to another large joint, such as the shoulder or knee **(Fig. 7-5)**.

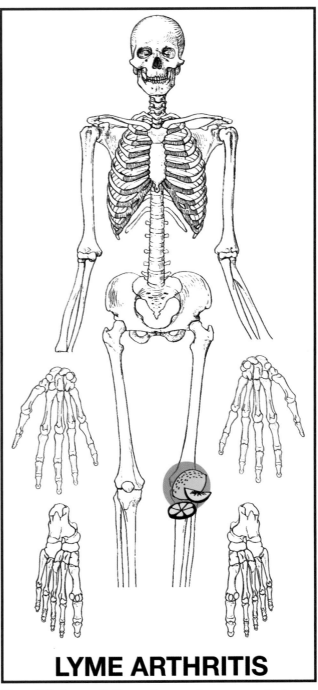

**Figure 7-5.** *Lyme arthritis usually presents as a monoarticular inflammatory arthritis, particularly in the knee.*

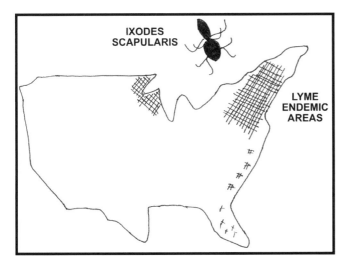

**Figure 7-4.** *Endemic areas for Lyme disease across the United States.*

### Diagnosis and Treatment of Lyme Disease

Prior to ordering tests for Lyme disease, the clinician needs to have a high suspicion for the disease, i.e. the patient should have visited a Lyme endemic area and the joint pain should be consistent with an inflammatory arthritis of the medium and large joints. Testing should be ordered with caution, as false positive results will cause confusion and delay the actual diagnosis.

The initial step in diagnosing Lyme disease is an enzyme-linked immunosorbent assay (ELISA), which tests for IgM and IgG antibodies to Lyme, indicating previous exposure. If the ELISA is positive, then a confirmatory Western blot test is done. If either of these is negative, then the patient should not be considered to have Lyme disease.

Treatment consists of antibiotic therapy with doxycycline or ceftriaxone, depending on the severity of infection.

### *Whipple's Disease*

*Whipple's disease* is a rare (about 1 in a million people), multi-system granulomatous infectious disease caused by the bacterium *Tropheryma whipplei,* which may present initially as joint pains of unknown etiology.

The classic history of *T. whipplei* infection is a middle-aged male with a long history of arthralgias (non-inflammatory joint pain, no joint swelling, no joint warmth), who later develops chronic diarrhea and weight loss. These symptoms can be present for years prior to diagnosis. Other systems may include endocarditis or CNS involvement with confusion and cognitive decline.

Patients with Whipple's disease may also have unique ocular findings, including *oculofacial-skeletal myorhythmia (OMM)*. This difficult-to-pronounce clinical finding consists of pendular nystagmus (up-down or left-right sinusoidal movements) of the eyes associated with contraction of the masticatory muscles.

Besides OMM, Whipple's has a classic triad of clinical findings that, if noted, are highly specific for the diagnosis:

- *Supranuclear ophthalmoplegia*: The patient cannot move the eyes in certain directions, usually up and down.
- *Dementia-cognitive decline*
- *Myoclonus*, a rapid, involuntary spasm of a group of muscles (e.g. the right arm rapidly jerks upwards, then goes back to rest)

Diagnosing Whipple's disease is difficult but needs to be on the physician's differential of unexplained joint pain in a middle-aged man. Most patients will not have the unique ocular findings but will present with prolonged arthralgias and weight loss. For diagnosis, most commonly a duodenal biopsy is performed; the organism can be seen with periodic acid-Schiff staining (PAS).

# Viral Causes Of Inflammatory Arthritis

A number of viral infections cause inflammatory joint pain **(Fig. 7-9)**. The organism may physically be in the joint space, but it is unclear if the organism itself causes the destruction within the synovium. The inflammatory joint pain is likely an immune response to the infection (influx of lymphocytes, neutrophils, and macrophages), which possibly contributes to the joint pain and swelling more than the organism itself. The pathophysiology is incompletely understood.

### *Parvovirus B19*

*Parvovirus B19* is a DNA virus that is distributed throughout the globe. Most adults have antibodies to the virus, indicating past exposure, but are asymptomatic. Rarely, exposure can cause an inflammatory arthritis that mimics rheumatoid arthritis. Remember Parvovirus B19 as the viral infection presenting as an acute symmetric polyarticular inflammatory arthritis after exposure to children!

Parvovirus B19 can have multiple clinical manifestations, including aplastic anemia, rash, and acute inflammatory arthritis. The acute inflammatory arthritis in adults is polyarticular, involves small joints, and resembles rheumatoid arthritis (metacarpophalangeal and proximal interphalangeal joints) of the hands.

Classically, the adult patient presenting with acute parvovirus B19 received the infection from a toddler who also has the disease, although Parvovirus B19 manifests differently in toddlers. Toddlers present with erythematous cheeks (*slapped cheeks disease*) and rarely an inflammatory arthritis **(Fig. 7-6)**.

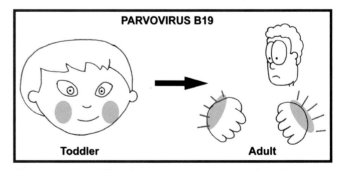

*Figure 7-6. In toddlers the most common presentation of Parvovirus B19 is reddened cheeks. In adults it can present as a polyarticular symmetric inflammatory arthritis that mimics rheumatoid arthritis.*

Confusingly, patients with acute parvovirus B19 often have a low-level rheumatoid factor positivity, which can lead the clinician to the incorrect diagnosis of rheumatoid arthritis. The major diagnostic clue is the timing. Patients with parvovirus B19 present more acutely with hand pain and recent exposure to an affected young child, whereas patients with rheumatoid arthritis present after a few months of daily pain that progressively worsens.

Another clue to the diagnosis is hematologic. Parvovirus B19 can present with a low hemoglobin and low white blood cell and platelet counts.

### Diagnosis and Treatment of Parvovirus B19

Parvovirus B19 can be diagnosed with serum IgM antibodies to parvovirus B19. The presence of IgM indicates recent infection. Most adults have IgG antibodies, indicating previous infection. Parvovirus B19 is a self-limiting disease, and the majority of patients begin improving within a few weeks to months without any intervention. NSAIDs can be given to treat the joint pain until it resolves.

## HIV

*HIV* is associated with a spectrum of rheumatologic conditions, including inflammatory arthritis and an inflammatory myopathy. These symptoms can be seen at any stage of HIV infection (acute or chronic). The course of HIV-related rheumatologic conditions has changed dramatically following the introduction of combination antiretroviral therapy. Inflammatory arthritis and inflammatory myopathy usually improve following the initiation of combination antiretroviral therapy.

## Hepatitis B

*Hepatitis B* is a double-stranded DNA virus that is common across the globe but uncommon where vaccination is available. Severe hepatitis can develop in patients infected with the virus through blood-borne contact (transfusion, IV drug use) or sexual contact.

Inflammatory arthritis can present as a prodrome prior to the development of acute hepatitis. Patients can have an inflammatory arthritis that involves the small joints of the hand (metacarpal phalangeal, proximal interphalangeal joints) and resembles rheumatoid arthritis.

The cause of the joint inflammation is immune complex deposition (the viral antigen attached to the antibody) in the synovial tissues. For unclear reasons, when immune complex deposition occurs, this activates the immune system (influx of lymphocytes, neutrophils, and macrophages) and the complement system. When the complement system is activated, the patient's serum complement 3 and 4 levels decrease as they are being actively deposited into the joint, which then activates more neutrophils into the area, leading to more inflammation. Many patients with immune complex disease will have a positive rheumatoid factor, which can confuse the diagnosis.

### Diagnosis of Hepatitis B

To diagnose hepatitis B, the patient, depending on the time of infection, will have a combination of positive hepatitis B serologies.

## Hepatitis C

Many patients with acute and chronic hepatitis C will develop extra-hepatic manifestations, including an inflammatory arthritis that can be polyarticular (resembling rheumatoid arthritis) or oligoarticular (usually involving the medium to large joints). As with hepatitis B, these patients may have a positive rheumatoid factor. One of the more important aspects of hepatitis C compared to other viral infections is the association of cryoglobulinemic vasculitis (see Chapter 13, Vasculitis).

## Chikungunya

This is a difficult-to-pronounce virus that sounds like chicken-gunya, so remember chickens hanging out in the Caribbean, where this disease is often contracted **(Fig. 7-7)**. Large outbreaks of this alpha virus have

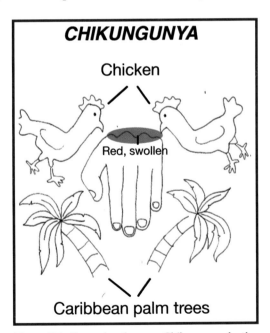

*Figure 7-7. Remember the name Chikungunya by the chickens pecking at the metacarpophalangeal joints, causing inflammation. Also notice the palm trees as this disease is often found in the Caribbean.*

occurred throughout Africa and Asia as well as the Caribbean, causing a symmetric polyarticular inflammatory arthritis that mimics rheumatoid arthritis.

Chikungunya is transmitted by *Aedes aegypti* mosquitos. The incubation period for the virus is 2-4 days, with the onset of an acute febrile illness with fever, arthralgia, myalgia, headache, and rash.

An inflammatory arthritis can occur that involves the small joints, usually a polyarticular symmetric inflammatory arthritis resembling rheumatoid arthritis.

Unfortunately, the joint pain can occur for up to 36 months, but usually lasts just a few months. There is no treatment for Chikungunya besides pain control.

## Ross River Virus

This is the most common mosquito-transmitted infection in Australia. The clinical presentation resembles Chikungunya (acute onset of polyarticular joint pain similar to rheumatoid arthritis). No treatment for Ross River virus is currently available; the goal of care is pain relief.

| FIGURE 7-8. BACTERIAL AND FUNGAL CAUSES OF INFLAMMATORY ARTHRITIS | | | | | | |
|---|---|---|---|---|---|---|
| | **Septic Bacterial Arthritis** | **Fungal Infections** | **Gonococcal Arthritis** | **Lyme Disease** | **Septic Joint from Myocobacteria** | **Whipple's Disease** |
| **Organism** | *Staphylococcus aureus* or *Streptococcus* species | • *Histoplasma capsulatum*<br>• *Cryptococcus neoformans*<br>• *Coccidioides immitis*<br>• *Candida species*<br>• *Sporothrix schencki*<br>• *Aspergillus fumigatus* | *Neisseria gonorrhoeae* | *Borrelia burgdorferi* | • *M tuberculosis*<br>• *M avium* complex<br>• *M kansasii*<br>• *M. marinum*<br>• *M abscessus*<br>• *M fortuitum*<br>• *M chelonae* | *Tropheryma whipplei* |
| **# of Joints** | Monoarticular rapidly worsening | Mono- or Oligo-articular, develops over days to weeks | Oligo-polyarticular, rapidly progressive but migratory | Mono-Oligoarticular: large joints, progresses over days to weeks | Mono-oligoarticular/ tenosynovitis, progresses over weeks to months | Oligo-polyarticular, progresses over months to years |
| **Synovial Cell Count** | Greater than 50,000 WBC/mm$^3$ | Between 10,000-50,000 WBC/mm$^3$ | Greater than 50,000 WBC/mm$^3$ | 2,000-100,000 WBC/mm$^3$ | 2,000-50,000 WBC/mm$^3$ | 2,000-50,000 WBC/mm$^3$ |
| **Important to know** | Needs to be ruled out in any acute inflammatory monoarthritis | Usually in immunocompromised patients. Importantly, *Sprothrix schenckii* occurs with exposure to gardening | Sexually active, young patient presenting with new onset inflammatory arthritis | Large joint inflammatory arthritis after exposure to ticks (hiking in the woods) | Slowly progressive inflammatory arthritis/ tenosynovitis usually in 1 joint but may spread to other joints. May develop painful swollen lymph nodes around site of inoculation. Remember *M. Marinum* is associated with salt water and fish tanks. | Middle aged man with long history of joint pains, presenting with diarrhea and weight loss |

| | FIGURE 7-9. VIRAL CAUSES OF INFLAMMATORY ARTHRITIS | | | | | |
|---|---|---|---|---|---|---|
| | **Parvovirus B19** | **Chikungunya** | **Ross River** | **Hepatitis B** | **Hepatitis C** | **HIV** |
| **Organism** | Immune response to Parvovirus | Possible Chikungunya viral invasion into synovial tissue in combination with immune response | Unclear if actual viral infection in the joint, or an immune response to the infection causes the inflammatory arthritis | Immune complex deposition vs actual hepatitis B deposition in synovium | Immune complex deposition | Likely an immune response associated with the virus; the HIV virus is usually not found in the synovial fluid |
| **# of Joints** | Polyarticular small joints | Polyarticular small joints | Polyarticular small joints | Oligo-polyarticular | Oligo-polyarticular | Oligo-polyarticular |
| **Synovial Cell Count** | 2,000-50,000 WBC/mm$^3$ | 2,000-50,000 WBC/mm$^3$ | 2,000-50,000 WBC/mm$^3$ | 2,000-50,000 WBC/mm$^3$ | 2,000-50,000 WBC/mm$^3$ | 2,000-50,000 WBC/mm$^3$ |
| **Important to know** | Acute onset rheumatoid arthritis-like symptoms, usually after contact with children | Acute onset rheumatoid arthritis-like symptoms after visiting the Caribbean, Asia, Africa | Acute onset rheumatoid arthritis-like symptoms after visiting Australia | In a patient with elevated liver enzymes; more common in areas without vaccination | Patient has a history of IV drug use, may have elevated liver enzymes | History of male to male sex, IV drug use, possibly with oral thrush and systemic symptoms like weight loss |

# 8

# *Autoinflammatory Disease*

*Autoinflammatory disease* is a different category than the other diseases in this book. Although autoinflammatory sounds similar to autoimmune, there are major differences.

*Autoimmunity* implies the immune system incorrectly identifies and reacts to its own body; this could be through antibodies or T cells interacting with the body's own tissues. Autoimmunity is thought to be an adaptive immune (B cell and T cells), as well as innate immune, system problem.

*Autoinflammatory*, in contrast, is not a problem of the body's *adaptive* immune system (B and T cells) recognizing its own body but a dysregulation of the body's *innate* immune system (neutrophils, macrophages, eosinophils, which are the first responders in the immune system). The theory is, the checks and balances of the body's innate immune system do not function properly, and the innate immune system will react when it's not supposed to. This reaction can cause a range of symptoms, such as fevers, rashes and possible inflammation within the joints (inflammatory arthritis). A prominent symptom that occurs in all of these diseases is fever, so a general term for this group of diseases is *periodic fever syndrome*.

## Periodic Fever Syndromes

*Periodic fever syndromes* differentiate themselves from autoimmune inflammatory conditions (rheumatoid arthritis, systemic lupus erythematosus) by being active at first and then, seemingly spontaneously, being inactive. A patient may feel completely normal, then feel very ill

within a few hours and be sick and feverish for days; then the symptoms spontaneously resolve. In between the flares, patients often feel completely normal, which can be for weeks or months depending on the disease. This contrasts with autoimmune diseases, which often have some level of involvement on a near-daily basis, although the severity can fluctuate from day to day.

The different periodic fever syndromes can be difficult to immediately distinguish, since they have similar presentations (consisting of fevers, arthralgias, and myalgias) when the disease is active. A helpful way to categorize the periodic fever syndromes are:

- Duration of fever
- Unique symptoms associated with the different fever syndromes

The different periodic fever syndromes and the unique aspects of each are discussed below. *Remember, all of these diseases have arthralgias and myalgias, so this is not mentioned in each description.* Also, whenever the periodic fever syndromes are active, the patient's inflammatory markers (Erythrocyte Sedimentation Rate, C-reactive protein) will be elevated. It is helpful to check inflammatory markers whenever an autoinflammatory syndrome is suspected, especially to see if the markers are elevated during a flare and then normalize between flares.

### Diagnosis of Autoinflammatory Diseases

The workup and diagnosis of each of the autoinflammatory diseases is discussed individually, but keep in mind that fever is usually the most prominent symptom a patient is experiencing, so infection needs to be ruled out as much as possible. Rheumatologists and infectious disease physicians should work together when evaluating these patients.

# Adult Onset Still's Disease (AOSD)

*Adult Onset Still's disease (AOSD)* is an inflammatory condition of unknown etiology. It is specifically referred to as *adult onset* because this is the adult form of systemic juvenile idiopathic arthritis (see Chapter 16, Pediatric Rheumatology).

*Daily fever.* The fever of AOSD classically occurs in the late evening, daily. In most cases, the fever resolves within a few hours, and the patient will be afebrile again for the remainder of the day until the next evening. This is termed a *quotidian* fever, which means daily fever. Once the fever occurs, the other symptoms discussed below usually follow. It is important to ask the patient what happens during the fever and between the fevers, as patients with AOSD often feel normal in between the fevers **(Fig. 8-1)**.

*Rash.* Classically a patient with AOSD will develop a fever in the late afternoon and subsequently develop a rash during the fever. The rash is often described as salmon-colored, flat and spotty, and presents on any body part. Usually the rash resolves when the fever resolves, so it is important to see the patient during the fever, or at least ask the patient to examine the skin while the fever occurs, since the patient may be unaware of the rash.

*Pharyngitis.* Pharyngitis is a unique symptom of AOSD; the patient will often describe a sore throat during the febrile period. This is thought to be due to inflammation of the cricothyroid cartilage.

## Diagnosis of AOSD

No diagnostic test exists at this time for AOSD, but certain lab values help make the diagnosis:

AOSD is associated with marked elevations in *serum ferritin.* Ferritin, a protein produced in the liver, can present as an *acute phase reactant* (a protein that rises during an inflammatory response), but in patients with AOSD the ferritin is often elevated both during and between the fevers, which makes it a useful test even when the patient isn't experiencing a disease flare. Also, the ferritin level can be markedly elevated, which helps guide the diagnosis. A normal ferritin level is between 40 to 200 ng/ml. In patients with AOSD, the number can exceed 3,000 ng/ml.

## Treatment of AOSD

Treatment of AOSD depends on the severity of disease. Mild disease may be treated with as needed

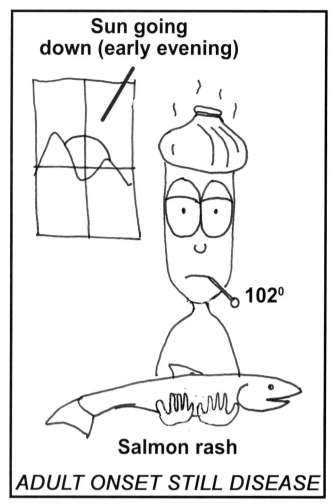

**Sun going down (early evening)**

**102⁰**

**Salmon rash**

*ADULT ONSET STILL DISEASE*

**Figure 8-1.** *Adult Onset Still's Disease with salmon-colored rash and quotidian fever.*

colchicine or NSAIDs like ibuprofen. More persistent disease can be treated with inhibition of interleukin-1 therapy: anakinra, canakinumab, or rilonacept.

## Important Complications of AOSD

*Macrophage Activation Syndrome (hemophagocytic lymphohistiocytosis [HLH])* is an important complication to be aware of in patients with AOSD. Macrophage activation syndrome is a hematologic condition that presents with bone marrow failure (low red blood cells, white blood cells, and platelets). Bone marrow biopsy reveals macrophages consuming hematologic cells (hence the "hemophagocytic" in the name).

Clues to macrophage activation syndrome occurring in a patient with AOSD:

- Low white blood cell count (*leukopenia*). Patients with active inflammation, as occurs with AOSD, have elevated white blood cell counts, so a low white blood cell count should raise suspicion for macrophage activation syndrome.

- High CRP but a *low* erythrocyte sedimentation rate; in contrast, in AOSD, both the CRP and the erythrocyte sedimentation rate are generally elevated.

# Familial Mediterranean Fever

*Familial Mediterranean Fever (FMF)* is an inherited autoinflammatory disorder, and, as the name suggests, is more common in people of Mediterranean ancestry. FMF is the most common of all the periodic fever syndromes.

FMF usually manifests in early childhood, but adult cases do occur. The characteristics of FMF are:

*Fever.* The fever of FMF is usually persistent, lasting 1-3 days before spontaneously resolving.

*Peritonitis.* Inflammation of the abdominal peritoneum, which produces rebound tenderness, guarding, and rigidity that looks like appendicitis. In fact, a diagnostic clue to FMF is that the patient previously had the appendix removed, but the appendix was normal.

*Pleuritis.* Inflammation of lung pleura, producing chest pain that is worse with breathing in.

## Diagnosis of FMF

FMF is caused by a mutation in the MEFV gene, which encodes a protein *pyrin,* which is involved in the production of interleukin-1. The mutations in the MEFV gene are thought to cause hyperexcitability of the pyrin protein and increased production of the pro-inflammatory cytokine, interleukin-1. Genetic testing can be performed on patients suspected of having FMF.

## Treatment of FMF

*Colchicine* is useful in FMF and is usually adequate for treating patients with infrequent attacks.

Targeted therapy for persistent disease is interleukin-1 inhibition with anakinra, canakinumab, or rilonacept.

## Important Complications of FMF

*Amyloidosis* is an important complication in patients with long-standing FMF. Amyloidosis is the inappropriate deposition of certain proteins in tissues, such as the kidneys. Amyloidosis occurs in patients with chronic inflammatory conditions, where the body is constantly producing proteins involved with inflammation. These proteins over time can deposit in organs and cause organ dysfunction. For reasons that aren't clear, patients with FMF appear to have a greater propensity to develop amyloidosis than other inflammatory conditions.

# Tumor Necrosis Factor Receptor-1 Associated Periodic Syndrome (TRAPS)

*TRAPS* is a rare autosomal dominant, autoinflammatory condition usually presenting within the first 10 years of life but rarely can present in early adulthood. TRAPS is caused by a mutation in the TNFRSF1A gene which provides instructions for production of tumor necrosis factor (TNF) receptor. The mutated receptor protein then clumps together in cells and allows for increased levels of the TNF cytokine, which triggers an inflammatory cascade.

*Fevers.* The fevers of TRAPS are long-lasting (5 days), occurring every 5-6 weeks.

*Ocular symptoms.* TRAPS involves the eyes more than other periodic fever syndromes, with many patients developing conjunctivitis and periorbital edema **(Fig. 8-2)**.

## Diagnosis of TRAPS

When the diagnosis is suspected based on the pattern of fevers and clinical symptoms, genetic testing can be done to evaluate for mutations in the TNFRSF1A gene.

## Important Complications of TRAPS

Amyloidosis is also a complication of a multiple-year history of TRAPS.

## Treatment of TRAPS

TNF inhibitors have been shown to be helpful in treating TRAPS. Interleukin-1 inhibitors, anakinra,

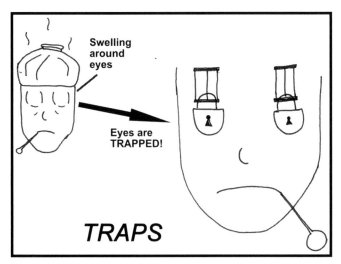

*Figure 8-2. Tumor Necrosis Factor Receptor-1 Associated Periodic Syndrome with fever and periorbital edema.*

canakinumab and rilonacept have also shown promise in treating TRAPS.

# Hyperimmunoglobulin D Syndrome

*Hyperimmunoglobulin D syndrome* usually presents in infancy, usually in patients of French or Dutch ancestry.

*Fevers.* The fevers of hyperimmunoglobulin D syndrome are long lasting, up to 4-7 days persistently.

*Lymphadenopathy.* The patient will usually develop palpable lymphadenopathy during the febrile episodes, more commonly in the cervical neck region.

*Peritonitis.* Peritoneal inflammation can also occur, causing abdominal pain similar to the pain seen in FMF.

## Diagnosis of Hyperimmunoglobulin D Syndrome

As the name suggests, hyperimmunoglobulin D syndrome involves elevated serum immunoglobulin D levels, as well as serum immunoglobulin A. The immunoglobulin levels continue to be elevated between attacks, which can help establish the diagnosis. Genetic testing can also be done to confirm the diagnosis, evaluating for mutations in the mevalonate kinase gene (MVK gene).

## Treatment of Hyperimmunoglobulin D Syndrome

NSAIDs, colchicine, glucocorticoids. Targeting interleukin-1 with anakinra, canakinumab, or rilonacept has shown to be effective in treating hyperimmunoglobulin D syndrome.

# Cryopyrin-Associated Periodic Syndromes (CAPS)

Three different diseases are considered among *CAPS*. All of them have mutations of the same NLRP3 gene, which encodes *cryopyrin*. Cryopyrin is a protein required for the secretion of interleukin-1 (IL-1), which triggers macrophage activation and recruitment of innate immune cells (macrophages, neutrophils, basophils). The CAPS pathophysiology is likely secondary to aberrant production of IL-1, triggering an inflammatory cascade.

*Rash.* Urticarial (hives) rash is the typical skin manifestation of CAPS. The three CAPS diseases:

1. **Familial Cold Autoinflammatory Syndrome (FCAS)** is the mildest form of CAPS. Patients develop fevers, rash, and conjunctivitis within 1-3 hours of cold temperature exposure. Unique feature: history of cold exposure prior to symptom development.

2. **Muckle-Wells Syndrome (MWS)** is the intermediately severe CAPS. Like other periodic fever syndromes, patients with MWS develop fevers (lasting 12-36 hours), rash, and joint pain. MWS usually presents in adolescence or early adulthood. A defining symptom of MWS is progressive *sensorineural hearing loss*. Sensorineural hearing loss is loss of function of the sensory nerves involved in hearing, in contrast to conductive hearing loss, which occurs from dysfunction somewhere in the ear canal (e.g. middle ear infection or obstruction of the external ear canal) **(Fig. 8-3)**.

3. **Neonatal-onset Multisystem Inflammatory Disease (NOMID)** is the most severe form of CAPS. It arises within the first months of life and is clinically characterized by recurrent fever, chronic aseptic meningitis, hives-like rash, and joint swelling. NOMID also has some combination of the other cryopyrin-associated periodic syndromes, e.g. cold exposure may worsen symptoms and

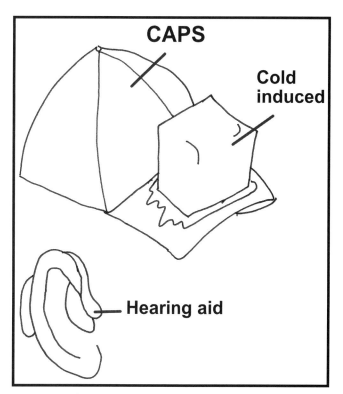

*Figure 8-3.* Cryopyrin-Associated Periodic Syndromes (CAPs). Remember that the patient can have autoimmune hearing loss (hearing aid) and rashes associated with cold exposure (ice cube).

sensorineural hearing loss may develop. NOMID is often fatal.

The 3 CAPS are thought to represent a continuum of the same disease process. Thus, there is overlap from one disease to another. For instance, FCAS may develop sensorineural hearing loss as seen in MWS.

## Treatment of CAPS

Considering that CAPS involves excess production of IL-1, the logical treatment is to block IL-1. Blocking IL-1 is accomplished with the medications anakinra, canakinumab, or rilonacept.

# Cases

1. HISTORY: A 25-year-old man develops a 3-month history of nightly fevers, sometimes up to 102° F. When he has the fevers, he develops joint and muscle aches, sore throat, as well as a faint, red/pink rash on various parts of his body. He feels no pain or discomfort between these episodes. He's had a thorough infectious disease workup, which was unremarkable.
LABORATORY: Reveals very high ferritin level as well as elevated ESR and CRP.
DIAGNOSIS: His history is consistent with the diagnosis of Adult Onset Still's Disease. His fever is daily towards the evening, accompanied by a red/pink rash and his labs reveal an elevated ferritin.
TREATMENT: Considering he is otherwise doing well, an initial treatment strategy in this case would be daily Non-Steroidal Anti-Inflammatory (NSAID) medication like naproxen or ibuprofen. If this doesn't help, then daily colchicine or low-dose daily glucocorticoid can be attempted.

2. HISTORY: The same patient presents 4 years later. His previous symptoms of fever and joint pains had resolved on daily colchicine. In the last few months, however, he has developed more fatigue and well as fevers. These fevers aren't the same as they were before. This fever is more constant throughout the day.
LABORATORY: Low white blood cell count, as well as a low erythrocyte sedimentation rate but very elevated CRP.
DIAGNOSIS: His symptoms do not sound consistent with his previous Adult Onset Still's Disease. His fever is now throughout the day, and he feels generalized fatigue. Adult Onset Still's is usually more of an episodic disease, with patients feeling normal in between flares. His labs are concerning because of the low white blood cell count and low erythrocyte sedimentation rate but elevated CRP. This pattern of labs and his history of Adult Onset Still's suggest macrophage activation syndrome.
TREATMENT: This patient should be hospitalized and undergo hematologic evaluation and bone marrow biopsy.

3. HISTORY: An 18-year-old woman from Greece presents with a multiple-year history of fevers, chest pain, and abdominal pain. She remembers being hospitalized as a child for these symptoms, and she had her appendix taken out at the time. Within a few months of the surgery, she had additional episodes that came and went. She feels her episodes of fevers are becoming worse, and not only does she get abdominal pain, but she also gets chest pain now that makes it painful to breathe in deeply. These episodes last 2-3 days at a time and then completely resolve, and she feels well.
DIAGNOSIS: This patient's symptoms are consistent with the diagnosis of Familial Mediterranean Fever.
TREATMENT: Daily colchicine should be initiated to lessen the risk of further attacks and lessen the risk of developing amyloidosis. If episodes persist despite maximizing doses of colchicine, then consider medications that block interleukin-1.

| | Adult Onset Still's (AOSD) | Familial Mediterranean Fever (FMF) | Tumor necrosis factor receptor-1 associated periodic syndrome (TRAPS) | Hyperimmunoglobulin D syndrome | CAPS | | |
|---|---|---|---|---|---|---|---|
| | | | | | FCAS | MWS | NOMID |
| **Fever** | Once a day, usually in the evening | 1-3 days continuous | 5 days continuous | 4-7 days continuous | 1 day | 12-36 hours | days |
| **Associated Symptoms** | Salmon colored rash, sore throat | Abdominal pain, chest pain | *Eyes*: conjunctivitis, periorbital edema *Joints*: focal extremity myalgias/ arthralgias | Cervical lymphadenopathy, abdominal pain | Urticaria with cold exposure | Urticarial rash, hearing loss | Urticarial rash, conjunctivitis, joint swelling |
| **Labs** | High ferritin | Elevated inflammatory markers | Elevated inflammatory markers | High levels of immunoglobulin D and A | Elevated inflammatory markers | | |
| **Gene** | Unknown | MEFV gene | TNFR1 gene | Mevalonate kinase gene (MVK) | NLRP3 encoding cryopyrin, excess production of IL-1 | | |
| **Complications** | Macrophage Activation Syndrome | Amyloidosis | Amyloidosis | | | Permanent hearing loss | Permanent hearing loss, death |

**FIGURE 8-4 PERIODIC FEVER SYNDROMES**

*CAPS*= Cryopyrin-Associated Periodic Syndromes; *FCAS=Familial Cold Autoinflammatory Syndrome; MWS=Muckle-Wells Syndrome; NOMID=Neonatal-onset multisystem inflammatory disease*

# Part III. Non-Inflammatory Arthritis

Non-inflammatory arthritis is by far a more common cause of joint pain than inflammatory arthritis. Trauma such as a sports injury resulting in a rotator cuff tear is considered non-inflammatory. (Although an inflammatory response will result from a torn muscle, the primary process isn't the immune system attacking the joint, so it's not considered an inflammatory arthritis.) Besides trauma, there are two very common causes of joint pain that you should know about: *osteoarthritis* and *fibromyalgia*.

# 9

# *Osteoarthritis*

*Osteoarthritis* is the most common cause of joint pain in the general population. Most people will be affected by osteoarthritis in some form if they live long enough. Osteoarthritis goes by many different names, such as *degenerative joint disease* and *wear-and-tear arthritis.* Osteoarthritis is a non-inflammatory cause of joint pain, meaning the immune system isn't the cause of the joint pain. Osteoarthritis manifests as a loss of cartilage between joints, which decreases joint space, along with the accumulation of bony outgrowths *(osteophytes),* which can rub against structures during joint movement, causing pain and a grinding sensation.

For unclear reasons, osteoarthritis has a predilection for certain joints **(Fig. 9-1):**

- Distal interphalangeal (DIP)
- Proximal interphalangeal (PIP)
- Thumb carpometacarpal (CMC) joints of the hands
- Knees
- Hips

Osteoarthritis can be divided into primary osteoarthritis and secondary osteoarthritis:

*Primary osteoarthritis* commonly occurs after age 50. It most often occurs in the finger (DIP) joints and thumb CMC joint, spine, hips, and knees.

*Secondary osteoarthritis* occurs from abnormal mechanical loading of a joint, e.g. one leg shorter than the other, which causes an abnormal gait with increased load on one hip. This may then result in cartilage loss and osteoarthritis. Trauma to a joint can also produce early osteoarthritis.

## History and Physical Exam in Osteoarthritis

### Hand Involvement in Osteoarthritis

Classically, the joints most affected by osteoarthritis are the *DIPs of the hands.* When an older patient presents with DIP joint pain, osteoarthritis is by far the most common cause. The examiner will notice bony enlargement of the DIPs *(Heberden's nodes)* as well as the PIPs *(Bouchard's nodes)* **(Fig. 9-2).** The joints will be hard on palpation in contrast to the soft, spongy feel in inflammatory arthritis. The patient may also complain of pain at the base of the thumbs (CMC joint), where the examiner may notice an enlargement *(squaring of the CMC joint)* **(Fig. 9-3).** The joint pain caused by arthritis worsens the more the patient uses the joint. There may be pain and weakness on opening jars or turning a doorknob.

### Knee Involvement in Osteoarthritis

*Knee osteoarthritis* is common in patients 50 years or older. It presents as a slowly progressive aching sensation in the knees, usually bilateral, but the pain can be worse on one side. The patient may complain of a cracking sensation in the knees; the pain worsens the more the patient uses the knees. The pain is especially pronounced going up and down stairs or getting out of a car. On physical exam, the examiner, with hand placed on the patient's knee, notes a cracking/popping

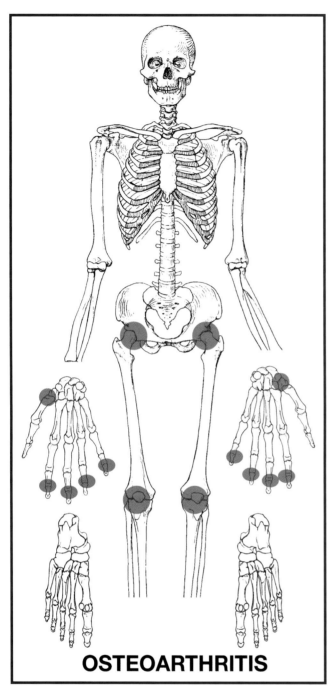

**Figure 9-1.** *Osteoarthritis. Symmetric joint pain in the small joints of the hands. The distal interphalangeal joints are most commonly involved. In the large joints, the hips and knees are most commonly involved.*

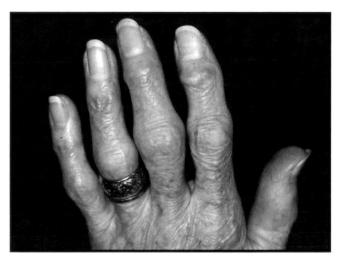

**Figure 9-2.** *Bouchard and Heberden's nodes. Notice the bony enlargement.*

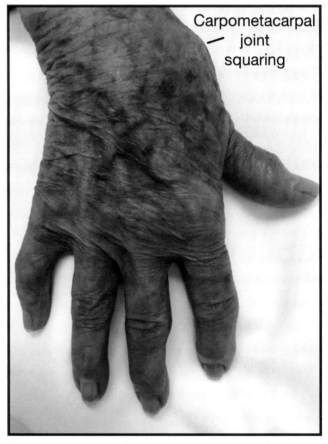

**Figure 9-3.** *Enlargement of the carpometacarpal joint in osteoarthritis, causing the area under the thumb to bulge outwards.*

(*crepitus*) sensation under the hand when repeatedly flexing and extending the knee.

*Hip Involvement in Osteoarthritis:* Osteoarthritis has a predilection for the hips and is the most common cause of hip replacement surgery. Most commonly, a patient complains of pain on ambulation, with pain radiating to the groin. This is important: hip pathology causes groin pain during movement of the hip joint.

## Laboratory and Imaging in Osteoarthritis

*Labs.* There are no lab tests for osteoarthritis.

*Imaging.* Four x-ray findings are consistent with the diagnosis of osteoarthritis **(Fig. 9-4)**:

1. *Narrowed joint space*, usually asymmetrically narrowed by loss of cartilage between the joints.
2. *Osteophytes* (bony outgrowths). Joints should glide past one another without interruption; osteophytes may collide during joint movement and produce a crepitus sensation (the sensation of cracking and popping).
3. *Subchondral sclerosis* appears as an increased density (whitening on x-ray) of bone immediately below the cartilage (subchondral).
4. *Subchondral cysts* are small circular-appearing lucencies in the bone immediately next to the cartilage.

## Differential Diagnosis of Osteoarthritis

*Hemochromatosis* is an important mimic of osteoarthritis. Hemochromatosis is a genetic disease of iron overload that affects multiple organ systems, including the liver and musculoskeletal system. A clue to the diagnosis of hemochromatosis is osteoarthritis of the second and third metacarpophalangeal (MCP) joints of the hand. Osteoarthritis normally affects the DIP and PIPs of patients, so the presence of osteoarthritis in these MCPs should prompt consideration for hemochromatosis.

*Pseudogout* (Calcium Pyrophosphate Dehydrate Disease—CPPD) is a crystalline disease that can cause pain in the hands in elderly patients. The pain may occur daily, or it may come and go over the course of days or weeks. A clue to the diagnosis is calcium deposition seen on x-ray (*chondrocalcinosis*) of the hands (see Chapter 6, Crystal Arthritis).

## Treatment of Osteoarthritis

Osteoarthritis is the most common cause of joint pain in the elderly and, frustratingly, is one of the causes of joint pain that we can do the least about. As of this writing, there are no medications that stop the progression of osteoarthritis or reverse the course of the joint space loss. Non-Steroidal Anti-Inflammatory Drugs (NSAIDs) help relieve pain caused by osteoarthritis, but they do not treat the underlying disease process or decrease disease progression. Physical therapy is employed to strengthen the muscles around the joint with the idea that stronger muscles will increase joint stability, lessen disease progression, and decrease pain. Intra-articular steroid injections are also used in osteoarthritis and can be effective for treating pain, especially in early disease.

It is not clear why intra-articular steroids give relief to patients with osteoarthritis, but the theory is that grinding produced by the abnormal proximity of one bone to another may produce a mild inflammatory response that will decrease with steroids. Any joint can be injected, but the smaller the joint (such as the joints in the hand), the more difficult it is to inject adequate amounts of steroid.

Many other medications have been made to inject into joints to treat osteoarthritis but lack data on their efficacy. Physical therapy and intra-articular steroid injections are used in an attempt to delay joint replacement surgery, which is the more definitive therapy for severe osteoarthritis.

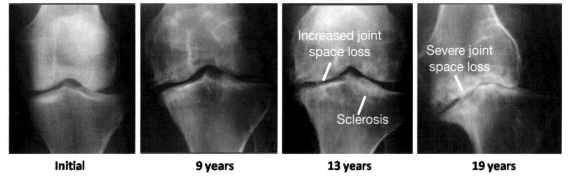

**Initial**      **9 years**      **13 years**      **19 years**

*Figure 9-4.* *X-ray image of the same knee over 19 years, showing progressive joint space loss (narrowing) as well as sclerosis around the joint (whitening of the edges). Image Courtesy of the American College of Rheumatology.*

# Cases

1. HISTORY: A 57-year-old man with no significant past medical history presents with a dull ache in his fingers (DIPs) as well as the base of his thumbs (CMCs). The pain worsens as the day progresses and when he does activities with his hands, like gardening. He feels the tips of his fingers are starting to point in different directions.

   DIAGNOSIS: This presentation is most consistent with osteoarthritis of the DIPs and thumb CMCs. As osteoarthritis progresses, the DIPs develop bony enlargements (*Heberden's nodes*), which can make the tips of the fingers look bent.

   TREATMENT: NSAIDs, physical therapy for the hand, or steroid injections into the joints. NSAIDs are appropriate for this patient as long as he has no history of kidney disease or gastrointestinal bleeding, which NSAIDs can worsen. NSAIDs would be the most practical, considering multiple joints are involved and the DIP joints are difficult to inject because of their small size. Another option would be NSAIDs in combination with injection of his CMC joints, which may provide 3-6 months of relief.

2. HISTORY: A 65-year-old man presents with a past medical history of chronic kidney disease and many years of osteoarthritis of his knees. He initially underwent physical therapy for the knees, which helped for many years, but then the pain progressed. He received knee injections every 4 months, which also helped initially, but now the pain is progressing.

   PHYSICAL EXAM AND IMAGING: His knees show no warmth, effusions, or tenderness to palpation. The range of motion of his knees is normal bilaterally, but crepitus is appreciated with the hand over the knees. X-ray shows complete joint space loss (bone-on-bone) of the knees bilaterally.

   TREATMENT: The patient cannot take NSAIDs because of his kidney disease. He has already undergone physical therapy as well as multiple injections without significant improvement. Total joint replacement is a reasonable option for this patient, and he should be referred to orthopedic surgery for evaluation.

# 10

# *Fibromyalgia*

*Fibromyalgia* is a chronic pain syndrome with a wide range of symptoms. There are multiple names used for fibromyalgia including *central sensitization* and *chronic fatigue syndrome*. The underlying pathophysiology of these conditions is not fully understood but is thought to be dysregulation of pain signaling within the brain. Fibromyalgia presents with a wide range of symptoms and can be difficult to treat, often resulting in patients being sent from physician to physician without anyone's taking ownership. It is important for physicians to recognize the diagnosis and empathize with a patient suffering with fibromyalgia.

Fibromyalgia is not an autoimmune disease, but is often seen by a rheumatologist because the patients are often young women with pain. It is important to rule out systemic autoimmune diseases so the appropriate treatment can be pursued.

## History in Fibromyalgia

Fibromyalgia presents over months to years with progressive diffuse body pain in both muscles and joints **(Fig. 10-1)**. The pain is described as a dull ache that worsens as the day progresses and with activity. These symptoms contrast with autoimmune inflammatory joint pain, which involves the joints, not the muscles; is worse in the morning; and usually improves with activity **(Fig. 10-2)**. Also, inflammatory arthritis usually involves certain joints, like the metacarpophalangeal joint (MCP) and not the distal interphalangeal

(DIPs) (or vice versa), whereas fibromyalgia will involve every joint in the hand.

Importantly, fibromyalgia is also associated with other kinds of symptoms:

- profound fatigue that significantly impacts daily life
- trouble falling asleep and staying asleep
- difficulty with concentration and word finding, often described as a "fibro fog"
- fluctuations in constipation and diarrhea a well as abdominal cramping
- anxiety and depression

It is unclear at the time of this writing why fibromyalgia occurs. Often the patient has an underlying depression and anxiety before the development of the diffuse pain and other symptoms. Sometimes the patient can pinpoint a past traumatic experience, whether personal or involving a loved one. The symptoms of fibromyalgia usually occur after months or years of stress, anxiety, or depression, or a combination of the three. Fibromyalgia likely has multiple causes. Chronic stress and anxiety may cause a maladaptive response of the brain and how it perceives signals, enhancing the perception of pain.

## Physical Exam in Fibromyalgia

Patients will often have pain diffusely with light palpation throughout the body. Palpating muscles on the upper arm or forearm should not elicit pain in an

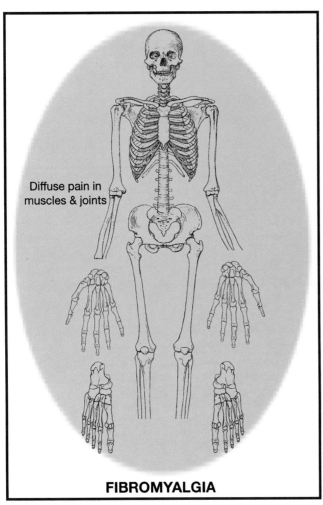

**FIBROMYALGIA**

*Figure 10-1. Fibromyalgia usually has an "all over the body" pain presentation.*

inflammatory condition (even inflammatory muscle diseases; i.e. *inflammatory myopathies* rarely have muscle pain) but will often elicit pain with fibromyalgia.

The *18 tender points* that were previously used for the diagnosis of fibromyalgia are no longer utilized for the diagnosis of the disease.

## Treatment of Fibromyalgia

Fibromyalgia is not autoimmune, but it can coexist with many other chronic health conditions that cause stress or anxiety. It is critical to recognize fibromyalgia, especially if the patient also has an underlying systemic autoimmune disease, such as systemic lupus erythematosus (SLE). If a patient with SLE has joint pain, it is important to distinguish the joint pain of SLE from that of fibromyalgia. If the SLE is active, the patient may require additional immunosuppression, but if immunosuppression is increased and the pain was caused by fibromyalgia, the pain will not improve and the patient will now be further immunosuppressed and more susceptible to infection.

Treatment of fibromyalgia is difficult, because the pathophysiology is poorly understood and may differ from patient to patient. Try to identify the cause of fibromyalgia, whether past trauma, severe anxiety, or depression. Antidepressant medications can help the symptoms if the underlying cause is depression or anxiety or a combination of the two. Mild exercise therapy can benefit patients with fibromyalgia, e.g. yoga, tai-chi, or water therapy.

Another critical aspect of fibromyalgia is the patient's accepting the diagnosis. Often, prior to making the diagnosis, the patient has been passed from specialist to specialist and has received an extensive and expensive workup. When you're confident in the diagnosis, it can be a major turning point in the care of the patient, as the workup can be stopped and the focus can be on finding ways to help the patient feel better.

## Case

HISTORY: A 33-year-old woman with a prolonged history of depression and anxiety presents with diffuse body pain. She first noticed the pain in her teens, and she feels it's slowly getting worse. The pain is an aching/

| FIGURE 10-2. FIBROMYALGIA VS AUTOIMMUNE INFLAMMATORY ARTHRITIS | | |
|---|---|---|
| | **Fibromyalgia** | **Autoimmune Inflammatory Arthritis** |
| **Area of pain** | Both muscles and joints | Joints |
| **Swelling** | No swelling | Swelling |
| **Timing** | Worse as the day progresses; worse with activity | Worse in the morning; better with activity |
| **Associated symptoms** | Fatigue, depression, anxiety, sleeping difficulties, concentration difficulties, fluctuation between constipation and diarrhea | Fatigue when the disease is active |

cramping sensation that worsens throughout the day. If she does too much work, like cleaning her house, she will have severe pain the rest of the day, and it can last for days. Accompanying the pain, she has severe fatigue, concentration and word finding difficulties, and difficulty falling and remaining asleep. She works as a secretary, and she's having trouble keeping track of tasks.

She is frustrated because she has been to multiple specialists, and nobody can give her an answer. She had "tons of lab tests," but all of them were normal.

PHYSICAL EXAM: There is diffuse pain to palpation throughout the body, muscles, and joints. No swelling or warmth is noted on examining the joints. Her muscle strength is intact.

DIAGNOSIS: Fibromyalgia

TREATMENT: The first step in treating this patient is recognizing the disease and empathizing with her. Validate her concerns and discuss how fibromyalgia can make people feel very poorly from a pain perspective, but it can also be debilitating from the fatigue and deficiency in cognitive function. Discuss various strategies for treating the pain and fatigue, such as mild yoga and undergoing physical therapy in a pool (water therapy). If this doesn't help in 3-4 months, you can try medications such as antidepressants. Explain to the patient that fibromyalgia is poorly understood, but hopefully every year we'll gain a better understanding of it and have better, more rapid treatment options.

# Part IV. Other Rheumatologic Diseases

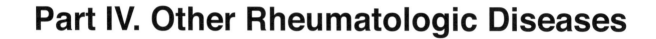

# 11

# Sjögren's Syndrome

*Sjögren's syndrome*, one of the more common autoimmune diseases, can cause significant discomfort but is rarely life-threatening. Like many autoimmune diseases, Sjögren's is more common in females than in males (9:1 ratio) with a prevalence of 1/1000 in the population. Uniquely, in Sjögren's syndrome the immune system's primary targets are the exocrine glands (salivary and lacrimal) as opposed to the joints, as in rheumatoid arthritis. This results in dry eyes from decreased tear production and dry mouth from decreased saliva. Sjögren's syndrome is commonly associated with joint pain and fatigue, making these symptoms part of the primary disease. Sjogren's syndrome is also associated with extra-glandular comorbidities, such as renal disease and neuropathies.

Many other autoimmune diseases also have dry eyes and dry mouth. The most common non-joint manifestation of rheumatoid arthritis is dry eyes and dry mouth. These patients are often described as having *secondary Sjögren's syndrome,* as opposed to primary Sjögren's syndrome, which is the topic of this chapter.

## History in Sjögren's Syndrome

The most common presentation is severe dry eyes and severe dry mouth. Joint pain and fatigue also accompany the eye and oral dryness in most cases.

### 1. Dry Eyes/Dry Mouth
- Severe dry eyes (*sicca* symptoms) to the point where the patient is using saline eye drops multiple times a day
- The dry mouth is often severe enough that patients carry water with them wherever they go. Salivary production is often low enough to allow increased bacterial growth in the mouth with a subsequent increase in cavities.
- Occasionally patients with severe Sjögren's syndrome have enlarged salivary glands and complain of a swollen face. The salivary glands enlarge from inflammatory cells (lymphocytes, neutrophils, and macrophages) that target the glands. On physical examination, the examiner may note parotid fullness to palpation.

### 2. Joint Pains
- Joint pain is common in Sjögren's syndrome, and is usually more of an arthralgia than an inflammatory arthritis. Arthralgia is a dull aching joint sensation that persists throughout the day, worse with activity, and not associated with swelling. This is in contrast with inflammatory arthritis, which has pain and swelling worse in the morning and improving with activity.
- The joint pain may respond to non-aggressive medications, such as non-steroidal anti-inflammatory medications or plaquenil, which is often used. More aggressive immunosuppression

does not appear to help the joint pain of Sjögren's syndrome.

### 3. Fatigue

- Fatigue is a major complaint in many patients with Sjögren's. Fatigue also accompanies active autoimmune diseases such as lupus and rheumatoid arthritis; however, fatigue seems more predominant in Sjögren's syndrome for unknown reasons.
- Immunosuppressive medications do not help the fatigue in Sjögren's syndrome, but patients usually benefit from mild physical therapy, such as yoga or water therapy.

## Other Extra-Glandular Manifestations of Sjögren's

The following manifestations of Sjögren's are less common but can have a high associated morbidity and mortality.

### 1. Malignancy

*B-cell lymphoma* is a major concern in Sjögren's syndrome. Most autoimmune diseases have a slightly higher risk of lymphoma compared to the general population, but the risk is much higher in Sjögren's for unclear reasons. The lymphoma usually develops in areas affected by Sjögren's, namely the parotid or submandibular glands. This may present as a persistent unilateral swelling of the face or jaw area. This can be difficult to discern from active Sjögren's syndrome, which also has facial glandular swelling; a clue to lymphoma may be unilateral swelling that persists. Sjögren's syndrome often has facial swelling, but it fluctuates with disease activity, so a patient may notice facial swelling one day that resolves in a few days. Persistent swelling should be biopsied to rule out lymphoma.

### 2. Kidney Disease

- *Renal Tubular Acidosis (RTA)* is an important manifestation of Sjögren's syndrome. Distal renal tubular acidosis occurs in a small percentage of patients with Sjögren's and is a reason to periodically check lab tests. A patient may have a low serum bicarbonate caused by the distal nephron's inability to excrete hydrogen ions; this leads to a buildup of hydrogen ions and subsequent metabolic acidosis (RTA). The kidney will also excrete more potassium, causing low serum potassium.
- Treatment for distal renal tubular acidosis is supplementation with oral sodium bicarbonate

tabs as well as potassium citrate to restore potassium levels.

### 3. Peripheral and Central Nervous System Dysfunction

- Nervous system involvement occurs in a minority of patients and usually causes annoying symptoms like a numb, tingling, or occasionally burning sensation in the extremities. But it can also develop into more serious complications, such as sensory and motor loss in the foot (*foot drop*) as well as spinal cord inflammation.
- Treatment of neurologic complications of Sjögren's depends on the severity of symptoms. If the patient has occasional pins and needles sensation in the arms, no aggressive immunosuppression is warranted. If there is persistent sensory loss or any motor loss, then consider using aggressive immunosuppression with high dose glucocorticoids.

### 4. Fetal Complications in Sjögren's

- Anti-SSA/SSB antibodies can cross the placenta in pregnant women, leading to fetal heart block. Pregnant patients with Anti-SSA/SSB antibody positivity need to be followed closely by a maternal-fetal obstetrics/gynecology doctor who specializes in high risk pregnancies. Plaquenil therapy given to the pregnant mother can decrease the risk of neonatal heart block.

## Physical Exam in Sjögren's Syndrome

- Ocular dryness can be difficult to estimate without an objective tool, like the *Schirmer's test*. Place a thin strip of special absorbent paper under the lower eyelid, wait 5 minutes, and then measure the length of wetness on the paper. An abnormal test is wetness less than 5 mm detected on the paper after 5 minutes (**Fig. 11-1**).
- Oral dryness can be evaluated by asking the patient to lift the tongue to the roof of the mouth; then evaluate the amount of salivary pooling at the base of the tongue. Quantitating salivary pooling is difficult, but a complete absence of saliva is consistent with Sjögren's syndrome.
- Joints are often mildly painful to palpation in patients with Sjögren's, but it is rare to see swollen, warm joints, as in rheumatoid arthritis.
- In patients with established Sjögren's, palpate for nodules in the parotid gland, neck, and axilla because the risk of lymphoma is higher than in the general population.

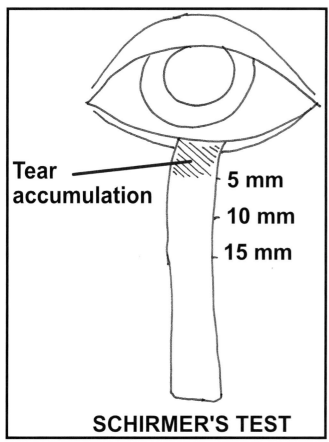

**Tear accumulation**

5 mm

10 mm

15 mm

**SCHIRMER'S TEST**

*Figure 11-1. Schirmer's test, showing the paper placed within the lower eyelid and measuring tear production by the progression of wetness on the paper.*

# Laboratory in Sjögren's Syndrome

Diagnosing Sjögren's syndrome can be difficult, since the symptoms of dry eyes, dry mouth, fatigue, and joint pain are fairly common in the general population, with most of these patients not qualifying for the diagnosis of Sjögren's syndrome.

The diagnosis of Sjögren's syndrome requires 2 out of the following 3:

*1. Antibody Testing*
- *Anti-SSA/SSB* antibodies are positive in most patients with Sjögren's, but can also be positive in systemic lupus erythematosus as well as a small fraction of the healthy population. The presence of Anti-SSA/SSB antibodies alone is not enough to make the diagnosis of Sjögren's syndrome.

*2. Objective Ocular or Oral Dryness*
- *Ocular Dryness:* The Schirmer's test mentioned above can be used to measure tear production. An ocular staining score can also be performed by an ophthalmologist. This test stains the patient's cornea and conjunctiva with fluorescein and yields a score based on how much of the dye gathers in these areas of the eye.
- *Oral Dryness:* Whole *sialometry* is an objective test to measure a patient's salivary production. The patient first spits out as much saliva as possible, then waits 5-15 minutes and spits into a pre-weighted cup; the saliva is then weighed. One variation of the test stimulates salivary production by applying citric acid swabs to the tongue. Normal results depend on how the test is performed.

*3. Tissue biopsy*
- The inner lip contains many minor salivary glands, which may show inflammation on biopsy. Biopsy is usually reserved for cases with high suspicion of Sjögren's syndrome and negative SSA/SSB serologies.

## Imaging in Sjögren's

MRI and ultrasound can show changes in the parotid gland structure consistent with Sjögren's syndrome, but these tests are non-diagnostic and are not part of the diagnostic criteria.

# Treatment of Sjögren's Syndrome

The treatment of the glandular manifestations (dry eyes and dry mouth) of Sjögren's syndrome can be frustrating. At this time we do not have medications that halt or reverse progression of the dryness. Many unsuccessful trials have tried aggressive immunosuppression to decrease inflammation in the secretory glands of the mouth and eyes—without success.

There are medications, though, that can treat the glandular symptoms of Sjögren's syndrome:
- Muscarinic agonists (e.g. *pilocarpine* and *cevimeline*) activate muscarinic receptors in the exocrine glands to stimulate saliva production and, to a lesser extent, tear production.
- Topical *cyclosporine* eye drops can increase tear production and limit the gritty sensation patients often complain of.

# Case

HISTORY: 27-year-old female presents with worsening oral and ocular dryness. She feels it started a few years previously, but now it's getting more annoying. She also feels her cheeks have become more swollen at times. Otherwise, she is feeling well besides some mild fatigue that has been present for the last few months.

PHYSICAL EXAM: Shirmer's test is performed, and only 2 mm of tear accumulation occurred over 5 minutes. Oral examination shows minimal salivary pooling underneath her tongue. Otherwise her physical exam is unremarkable.

LABORATORY: ANA is negative, but Anti-SSA/SSB are both positive.

DIAGNOSIS: Sjögren's syndrome. She has both laboratory evidence (Anti-SSA/SSB) as well as objective evidence of ocular dryness.

TREATMENT AND MONITORING: Advise the patient to be followed by ophthalmology to monitor eye health and discuss eye drop options. Muscarinic agonists can be attempted to see if the patient notices benefit from an oral dryness standpoint. She should also be followed closely by a dentist to watch for dental cavities. Considering the patient is within childbearing age, she needs to be aware of the potential for anti-SSA/SSB to travel across the placenta and cause fetal heart block. Plaquenil therapy is reasonable as this lowers the risk of placental transfer if she were to get pregnant.

Labs should be periodically checked, including serum potassium and bicarbonate levels to monitor for evidence of renal tubular acidosis. The patient should be aware of the increased risk of lymphoma and of the need to alert her physician to any new nodules she may feel on her body.

# 12

# *Scleroderma*

The word *scleroderma* means thick skin, which is the most predominant symptom of scleroderma. Scleroderma, also called *systemic sclerosis*, causes skin thickening, most predominately at the tips of the fingers, but can extend to the entire body. It can involve internal organs like the lungs and kidneys. The disease is rare with an estimated prevalence of about 0.03% of the population being affected.

Skin thickening, the cardinal symptom of scleroderma, starts at the tips of the fingers and progresses more proximally. The extent of thickening places the patient in either the *limited scleroderma* category (skin thickening of only the fingers and hands up to the wrist) or the *diffuse scleroderma* category (skin thickening throughout the body).

## Pathophysiology of Scleroderma

Scleroderma differs from the other diseases in this book because we tend to associate autoimmune diseases with inflammation, where tissue from a joint or muscle demonstrates various inflammatory cells (neutrophils, macrophages, lymphocytes), which damage the involved tissue. Scleroderma is different; it is not an overtly inflammatory disease but more of a progressive fibrotic disease. We think the immune system dysfunctions in a way that allows this fibrosis to occur, but presently the pathogenesis is incompletely understood. When fibrosis occurs in organ systems other than the skin, it can cause severe morbidity and mortality.

## History in Scleroderma

Scleroderma can affect multiple organ systems. When scleroderma is suspected, inquire about the following:

*Raynaud's phenomenon* is present in nearly every patient with scleroderma, but is also somewhat common in the general healthy population. Raynaud's phenomenon occurs when a person is exposed to cold and the digits (usually fingers, but toes as well as the tongue can be involved) turn different colors, classically white, then blue then red, with accompanying discomfort. What's occurring in the fingertips is disruption of blood flow (white) **(Fig. 12-1)** and transient ischemia of the tissue (blue), then resolution of disruption and subsequent increased blood flow (red). The severity of Raynaud's can range from an annoyance to extremely painful, causing digital ischemia and ulcerations at the tips of the finger from poor blood flow.

Raynaud's phenomenon can be divided into two categories: *primary* and *secondary* Raynaud's.

*Primary Raynaud's* is not uncommon in the general population and is idiopathic, meaning we don't think it is associated with an underlying autoimmune disease. Primary Raynaud's is usually noticed in young women in their early 20's. The patient notices a color change in the fingers when exposed to cold temperatures. The symptoms will last minutes, and then blood flow will return to normal. Primary Raynaud's is often more of an annoyance, and patients do not usually seek medical attention for it.

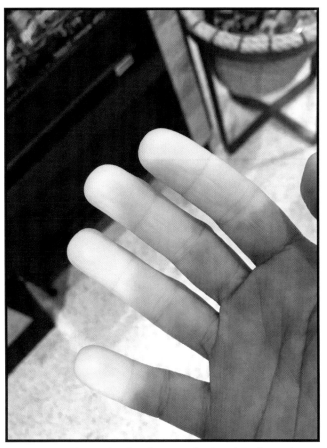

*Figure 12-1.* Dramatic color change at the tips of the fingers in Raynaud's phenomenon.

changes are usually more pronounced in between the distal interphalangeal joint (DIP) and the proximal interphalangeal joint (PIP) but can be seen throughout the entire finger. Skin thickening can be evaluated when the examiner pinches the skin on the dorsum of the finger. Normally a small tent of skin can be lifted from the finger, but in patients with sclerodactyly, the examiner cannot pull up loose skin (**Figs. 12-2, 12-3**).

*Telangectasias* are small (0.5-1mm in diameter) red lesions visible on the skin, most notably on the face. The lesions are caused by dilatation of the small blood vessels at the surface of the skin in patients with scleroderma, but they also occur in other conditions, such as liver failure.

*Nail fold capillaroscopy* can be done in the clinic if you have access to nail fold capillaroscopy or a source of light and magnification so you can visualize the capillary loops at the base of a patient's nail bed. In a normal healthy population, the capillaries will appear as visible loops at the base of the nails. They will be relatively homogenously dispersed and be about the same size. In patients with underlying scleroderma or other autoimmune disease, you may see dilated capillary loops (**Fig. 12-4**), or in severe disease you'll see patches where the capillary loops are no longer present (*dropout*). A patient who experiences Raynaud's phenomenon and has changes in the nail fold capillaries could have an underlying autoimmune disease.

## Categorizing Scleroderma

The extent of skin thickening on a patient's body defines the category of the disease, labeling the condition as either *limited* or *diffuse scleroderma*. The category of limited or diffuse is important to know because the different categories have different internal organ manifestations, as we shall discuss (**Fig. 12-5**).

*Limited scleroderma* means the skin thickening does not progress proximal to the forearm of the patient. The skin thickening is confined to the most distal areas of the extremities (fingers and toes). Patients with limited scleroderma are more likely to develop pulmonary

*Secondary Raynaud's* occurs in patients with an underlying autoimmune disease like scleroderma or dermatomyositis (many different diseases can have accompanying Raynaud's phenomenon). Secondary Raynaud's can be more severe than primary Raynaud's; the disruption of blood flow can become more permanent, leading to ulcerations of the tips of the fingers. Nailfold capillaroscopy can help distinguish between primary and secondary Raynaud's. In secondary Raynaud's, the patients often have abnormal nailfold capillaries. (See nailfold capillaroscopy below.)

*Esophageal dysmotility* is a common complaint in patients with scleroderma. The patient will often report food getting stuck in the throat.

*Gastro-Esophageal Reflux Disease.* The lower esophageal sphincter often does not contract in patients with scleroderma, allowing acidic contents from the stomach to move upwards into the esophagus, causing the symptoms of heartburn.

## Physical Exam in Scleroderma

*Sclerodactyly* refers to the finding of skin thickening and tightening in the fingers. The skin

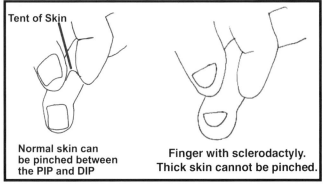

*Figure 12-2.* Sclerodactyly.

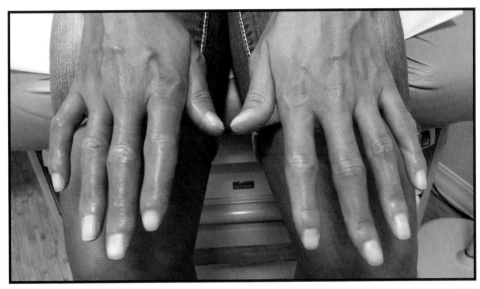

*Figure 12-3.* *Hands in a patient with scleroderma. Notice the shiny and tightened appearance of the skin on the fingers.*

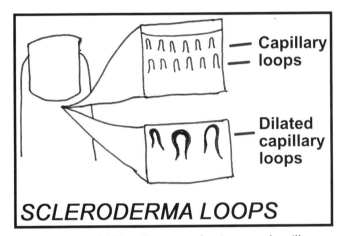

*Figure 12-4.* *Nail fold capillaroscopy, showing normal capillary loops compared to abnormal dilated capillary loops in a patient with scleroderma.*

hypertension (discussed below). Other complications associated with limited scleroderma are *calcinosis* (buildup of calcium under the skin, which can form painful nodules), *esophageal dysmotility* (patients may complain of swallowing difficulties), and *telangiectasias* (small capillary dilatations that can appear as red dots on the face or other skin surface). These manifestations are referred to as CREST syndrome: Calcinosis, Raynaud's, Esophageal dysmotility, Sclerodactyly, and Telangiectasias.

*Diffuse scleroderma* manifests as skin thickening more proximal than just the hands and can involve the skin throughout the body. Interstitial lung disease (fibrotic lung disease) is associated with diffuse scleroderma.

## Laboratory Tests in Scleroderma

Multiple antibodies are associated with scleroderma, but the following 3 are the most common and the ones to remember:

1. *Anti-centromere antibody* is associated with limited scleroderma.
2. *Anti-SCL70 (topoisomerase)* is associated with diffuse scleroderma and interstitial lung disease.
3. *RNA polymerase III* is the antibody that is most associated with scleroderma renal crises (see below) and rapidly progressive diffuse skin thickening.

Suspicion for scleroderma should be raised when you're evaluating a patient with sclerodactyly as well as a history consistent with Raynaud's phenomenon. As long as the skin thickening is not rapidly progressive (diffuse skin thickening in less than 5 months) the initial antibodies to order are *anti-centromere* and *anti-SCL70*. If either of them is positive, this confirms the diagnosis of

| FIGURE 12-5. LIMITED VS DIFFUSE SCLERODERMA | | |
|---|---|---|
| **Category of Scleroderma** | **Antibody** | **Disease Complications** |
| Limited scleroderma | Anti-centromere | Pulmonary hypertension |
| Diffuse scleroderma | Anti-SCL70 (topoisomerase) | Interstitial lung disease |
| | RNA-polymerase 3 | Scleroderma renal crises |

scleroderma. If the patient has rapidly progressive skin thickening (skin thickening throughout body over the course of 2-5 months), order the test for *RNA polymerase III*.

# Complications of Scleroderma

In many patients with scleroderma, the primary complaint is finger skin thickening with accompanying Raynaud's and possibly ulcerations at the tips of their fingers. Some distinct but rare complications that are also associated with scleroderma are important to recognize since they have high associated morbidity and mortality.

## Scleroderma Renal Crisis

In *scleroderma renal crisis*, the primary organ that is damaged is the kidney. It is not clear what triggers this, but rapid worsening of renal function occurs with associated acute elevations in blood pressure. The pathophysiology of the renal crisis is poorly understood. The blood vessels in the kidney develop multiple fibrotic layers, called *onion skinning*. These findings on renal biopsy are referred to as *thrombotic microangiopathy*, which you can see in other conditions such as very high blood pressure. While not a specific biopsy finding for scleroderma renal crisis, if you have these histologic findings in a patient with scleroderma, it is highly concerning for scleroderma renal crisis.

Another clue to the diagnosis of scleroderma renal crisis is acute anemia from *microangiopathic hemolytic anemia*, a type of red blood cell destruction in the small blood vessels. Blood smears should be done on these patients, which will reveal *schistocytes* (destroyed red blood cells).

Scleroderma renal crisis is more associated with diffuse skin disease compared to limited skin disease and usually occurs within the first 5 years of disease onset. Importantly, it is most associated with the antibody *RNA polymerase III*.

The treatment for scleroderma renal crises is the expeditious use of angiotensin-converting enzyme (ACE) inhibitors. This is one of the only instances in medicine where a patient with a rising creatinine will be treated with ACE inhibitors! Prior to the use of ACE inhibitors, patients with scleroderma renal crises frequently became dialysis dependent or died. ACE inhibitors are thought to be beneficial because the medication reverses the angiotensin II-induced vasoconstriction, which is greatly increased in scleroderma renal crises.

## Pulmonary Hypertension

*Pulmonary hypertension* is the lung manifestation that is most often associated with limited scleroderma and *anti-centromere* antibody positivity. Pulmonary hypertension is elevated blood pressure in the pulmonary artery as it exits the right ventricle. It is unclear why this occurs, but the same mechanism that involves the vessels of the fingers (Raynaud's phenomenon) is likely occurring in the pulmonary artery. This can cause shortness of breath and eventually lead to right-sided heart failure because the right ventricle becomes progressively dilated from the increased pulmonary artery pressure.

It is important for these patients to have pulmonary function testing as well as an echocardiogram that can estimate the right ventricular systolic pressure (a number above 45 mmHg can suggest pulmonary hypertension, but this is not diagnostic). The only way to diagnose pulmonary hypertension with certainty is a right heart catheterization, which measures a mean resting pulmonary artery pressure of greater than 25 mmHg in pulmonary hypertension.

## Interstitial Lung Disease

*Interstitial Lung Disease* is a category of lung disease in which the small airways become diffusely fibrotic from scarring that likely occurred from previous inflammation with subsequent abnormal healing. Interstitial lung disease can be idiopathic or associated with exposure histories (like asbestosis) or autoimmune conditions (like diffuse scleroderma). The pulmonary function tests and CT imaging of the chest will be abnormal in patients with interstitial lung disease.

Every patient with scleroderma, regardless of their antibody, should have a chest x-ray, an echocardiogram (evaluating for elevated right ventricular systolic pressure and pulmonary hypertension) and pulmonary function testing, which can give clues to underlying lung pathology, such as pulmonary hypertension or interstitial lung disease. To monitor for signs of scleroderma renal crisis, patients should have their blood pressure checked often, as well as their serum creatinine, as both will be elevated in scleroderma renal crisis.

# Differential Diagnosis of Scleroderma

Here are three important mimics of scleroderma:

- *Nephrogenic systemic fibrosis* is a disease that causes fibrosis of the skin and internal organs but is distinct from scleroderma because it is caused by exposure to *gadolinium contrast* while undergoing an MRI in a patient with renal insufficiency. This is a progressive condition without effective therapies and is one of the principle reasons patients with renal insufficiency are not given IV contrast with MRIs.
- *Morphea* is localized patches of skin thickening that can occur in any location on the body, including the face. To distinguish this from scleroderma,

in morphea the hands are not involved and the patient does not have Raynaud's phenomenon. The histology resembles scleroderma, and the skin thickening can progress to involve multiple parts of the body in patches.

- *Eosinophilic fasciitis* is a localized skin thickening, usually on the distal forearms of young patients. For unknown reasons, there is an association with strenuous exercise prior to developing the skin thickening. Think of *eosinophilic fasciitis* when you see a young patient with localized skin thickening of the forearms, not involving the fingers, with no associated Raynaud's. A big clue to the diagnosis is eosinophilia in the blood.

# Treatment of Scleroderma

Unfortunately, scleroderma is a disease with a long list of drug trials with a variety of immunosuppressant medications, but none have shown efficacy in reversing the disease. The important aspect of managing these patients is recognizing and treating secondary organ damage, such as pulmonary hypertension or scleroderma renal crises.

Raynaud's with digital ulcerations can be treated with different strategies, including medications that dilate blood vessels, like calcium channel blockers, nitric oxide paste on the hands, or more aggressively with a phosphodiesterase type 5 inhibitor such as *sildenafil* (Viagra). Other medications are beneficial, such as *pentoxifylline*, which helps red blood cells maneuver through the blood vessels more easily. In patients with digital ischemia and high risk of losing a finger, prostaglandin analog *alprostadil* will help with vasodilation.

# Cases

1. HISTORY: A 37-year-old woman reports progressively worsening color changes in her fingers whenever she is exposed to the cold, with some associated pain at the tips of her fingers. She also occasionally notices some swallowing problems where she feels food gets stuck in her throat for a few seconds. She doesn't feel like she has any shortness of breath with exertion.
PHYSICAL EXAM: Notable for skin tightness at the tips of her fingers. You cannot pinch the skin close to the tips of her fingers.

DIAGNOSIS: Her symptoms are consistent with limited scleroderma, and the most likely antibody associated with her presentation is anti-centromere.
TREATMENT AND MONITORING: When evaluating a patient with scleroderma, it is important to document the organ involvement. A baseline cardiac echocardiogram should be obtained to evaluate for elevations in the right ventricular systolic pressure, which could indicate pulmonary hypertension. It is also important to have a gastroenterology evaluation to document dysphagia with eating. The patient can be given a low dose calcium channel blocker for her Raynaud's, and the dose can be increased over time, depending on how she tolerates it. (Her blood pressure may decrease dangerously, and she may develop dizziness or syncope on higher doses.)

2. HISTORY: A 42-year-old woman presents to the emergency room with a severe headache. She says her skin has rapidly thickened throughout her body over the last few months. She has severe color change and ulcers at the tips of her fingers. She also notes difficulty swallowing and severe heartburn.
PHYSICAL EXAM AND LABS: In the emergency room her blood pressure is found to be 210/120. She has diffuse skin thickening throughout her body, including her face. Her hemoglobin is low at 7.6 g/dl, and her creatinine is elevated at 4.5 mg/dl.
DIAGNOSIS: Her constellation of symptoms is concerning for scleroderma renal crisis. Her rapidly progressive skin thickening is consistent with anti-RNA polymerase III antibody, which is also associated with scleroderma renal crisis. Her hemoglobin is low because of microangiopathic hemolytic anemia, which damages small blood vessels, with subsequent tearing of the red blood cells. Blood smears will reveal schistocytes, which are torn red blood cells.
TREATMENT: ACE inhibitor medications should be used promptly to try to improve her kidney function and possibly avoid dialysis. *Captopril* is often used because it is given multiple times a day, and the dose can be up titrated if her blood pressure does not start decreasing. The patient may be eventually placed on dialysis from renal failure, but the ACE inhibitor should be continued for at least 6 months, because the kidney may recover even that long after the initial injury.

# 13

# Vasculitis

*Vasculitis* is an umbrella diagnosis referring to an inflammatory infiltration (macrophages, neutrophils, lymphocytes, eosinophils) within the walls of blood vessels. When this occurs, the walls of the blood vessels weaken and become aneurysms; or the walls can thicken, decreasing the amount of blood that gets through, with resultant organ ischemia. The different types of vasculitis are most commonly categorized by the size of the blood vessels involved, e.g. large vessel vasculitis involving the aorta, or medium vessel vasculitis involving the mesenteric blood vessels (blood supply to the intestines).

Vasculitis can be a difficult diagnosis to make. Many times there are no diagnostic lab tests, and sometimes the affected blood vessel can't be easily biopsied (at least without a possibility of severe harm to the patient). You need to rely on a combination of history, physical exam, and imaging modalities to make the diagnosis as best you can.

It is important to also understand that, like most of the diseases in rheumatology, we don't understand why these diseases happen and why certain blood vessels are involved when others are not. Vasculitis is a mysterious category of autoimmune disease, but luckily we are becoming better at diagnosing and treating it!

## Large Vessel Vasculitis

### Giant Cell Arteritis (Temporal Arteritis)

Giant Cell Arteritis (GCA, previously called *Temporal Arteritis*) is the more common form of vasculitis.

Physicians who work in primary care will inevitably encounter a patient suffering from the symptoms of GCA. GCA is a vasculitis of the large and medium-sized blood vessels, usually around the head and face and occurring almost exclusively in patients older than 50 years old; the majority of patients with GCA are in their 70's and 80's.

**History in Giant Cell Arteritis**

The *classic presentation* is an elderly patient complaining of new onset headache, jaw pain, and visual changes **(Fig. 13-1)**.

*Headache.* Consider GCA in an elderly patient with a new headache. The headache can involve any part of the head, but classically the temporal area. The patient may complain of pain with combing the hair or touching the temporal side of the head. The pain is caused by inflammation within the temporal artery, which is superficial on the sides of the head.

*Jaw claudication.* Patients may also describe jaw pain with eating (*jaw claudication*). The arteries of the jaw muscles become narrowed, and the jaw muscles can't get enough blood when they're used, so it's like angina of the jaw. It is important to differentiate other causes of jaw pain such as *temporal mandibular joint (TMJ)* disorder, which may cause pain at rest, opening the mouth, or biting down. TMJ disorder can occur in the elderly, who may have poorly fitted dentures.

*Ocular manifestations.* The most feared complication of GCA is *inflammation of the arteries of the eye*, which can lead to sudden, painless, and permanent blindness.

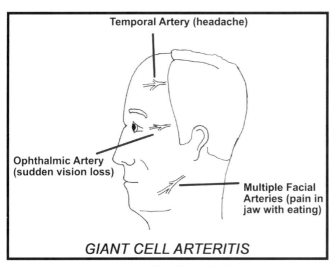

**Figure 13-1.** *Arteries involved in Giant Cell Arteritis.*

When GCA is suspected, ask the patient if any double vision or sudden vision loss has occurred.

### Physical Exam in Giant Cell Arteritis

The physical exam in GCA may be unrevealing, but there are a few areas to pay attention to:

*Temporal artery palpation.* The examiner can palpate and appreciate the temporal artery pulse in patients suspected of GCA. In active disease, palpation of the temporal artery is often painful. In severe disease, palpable nodules can be appreciated over the temporal artery.

*Four extremity blood pressure.* The aorta and its branches that supply the arms and the legs can be involved in GCA. If the blood pressure differs significantly between the arms or between the legs, this could indicate decreased blood flow to an extremity and possible vasculitis.

*Bruits.* If a large vessel such as the subclavian or femoral arteries has narrowing from vasculitis,the disruption to blood flow may produce a whooshing sound that is appreciated by the examiner placing a stethoscope over the blood vessel.

### Diagnosis of GCA

The only definitive way to diagnose GCA is with a temporal artery biopsy, a procedure where a small section of the artery is taken from the side of the head and evaluated by a pathologist under a microscope for evidence of inflammation in the vessel. Importantly, the biopsy is not a perfect test; GCA may involve *skip lesions* within the blood vessel, meaning some parts of the vessel are perfectly normal and then a millimeter away the vessel is actively inflamed. The biopsy may just capture a small portion of normal blood vessel tissue and miss the inflammation millimeters away.

If the biopsy result is positive for GCA, then you have a definitive diagnosis; but if the biopsy results are negative, and the patient's symptoms are highly suggestive of GCA, then treatment with glucocorticoids should be initiated regardless to prevent complications of GCA. Treatment with glucocorticoids is also important for the diagnosis; glucocorticoids should rapidly reduce the patient's symptoms. If the symptoms do not respond within 3-5 days, then GCA is less likely.

There is no blood test for GCA, but when the disease is active, the patient will have elevated inflammatory markers in the blood in 90% of the cases. Sometimes the Erythrocyte Sedimentation Rate will be as high as 100 mm/hr or more (see Chapter 17, Antibodies and Other Lab Tests). If symptoms are classic for GCA, normal inflammatory markers should not dissuade you from pursuing the diagnosis; rarely the markers will be normal in patients with active disease.

### Treatment of GCA

The good news is that GCA usually responds promptly to high dose glucocorticoids. If you suspect GCA (new temporal headaches, jaw claudication), promptly start the patient on prednisone to decrease the risk of developing permanent blindness. The patient should then get a temporal artery biopsy to confirm the diagnosis. Treatment should not be delayed while awaiting temporal artery biopsy, since the biopsy results will be positive for up to 2 weeks after initiating glucocorticoids.

*Interleukin-6* inhibition with *tocilizumab* has been shown to be effective in treating GCA. Tocilizumab should not be used by itself initially but in conjunction with glucocorticoids.

## *Polymyalgia Rheumatica*

*Polymyalgia rheumatica (PMR)* is a disease that is associated with Giant Cell Arteritis and is sometimes referred to as GCA Jr. PMR causes pain and stiffness in the shoulders and hips/upper thighs in patients over the age of 50. Pain is usually much worse in the morning, gets better as the day progresses, and is located proximally in the limbs (shoulders and upper thighs) **(Fig. 13-2)**, in contrast to other inflammatory conditions such as rheumatoid arthritis, which affect the hands and feet. Other conditions affecting proximal areas are the inflammatory myopathies (see Chapter 14, Inflammatory Myopathies), but remember that inflammatory myopathies present as proximal weakness and are generally painless, whereas the primary symptoms of PMR are pain and stiffness. PMR can involve the hands similar to rheumatoid arthritis,

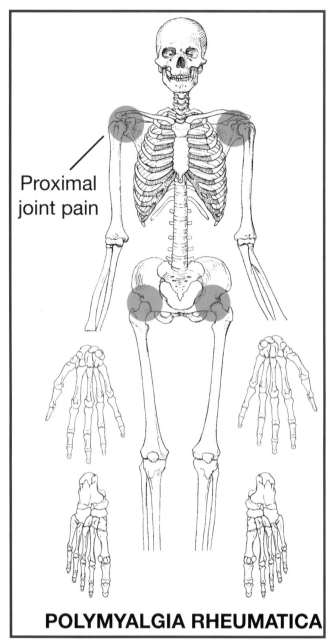

Proximal
joint pain

**POLYMYALGIA RHEUMATICA**

*Figure 13-2.* Proximal joint pain, shoulders and hips/thighs, pain and stiffness worse in the morning and better with activity.

but the predominant symptoms of pain and stiffness in PMR is the proximal muscle groups.

There is no diagnostic laboratory test for PMR, but the inflammatory markers are usually elevated, which can raise your suspicion for PMR. The diagnosis can be made by giving a low dose of prednisone; the patients with PMR often feel dramatically better within 24 hours. You will make many friends if you diagnose PMR, as the patients are usually feeling very frustrated by the pain and stiffness, and prednisone will make them feel "night and day" better.

PMR and GCA often coincide, but either disease can be seen alone. If a patient has been diagnosed with PMR, ask about symptoms of GCA. If GCA is being considered, and if the patient also has symptoms suggesting PMR, the likelihood of underlying GCA is much higher.

## Takayasu's Arteritis

*Takayasu's arteritis* is a large vessel vasculitis affecting a much younger population (ages teens-30s), with a propensity to affect the large vessels branching out of the aorta. In contrast, GCA is strictly seen in patients above the age of 50 years old and involves the arteries in the head, and occasionally the aorta. The classic patient demographic of Takayasu's arteritis is an Asian female somewhere between her teens and 30's, but it can occur in any ethnicity.

### History in Takayasu's arteritis

The first symptoms of Takayasu's arteritis are usually nonspecific: malaise, fevers, and joint pains similar to a prolonged viral illness. The disease then progresses to an overt vasculitis, usually of the aorta and its main branches, such as the subclavian, carotids, renal, and iliac arteries. Because of the large vessel involvement, the limbs are usually the most affected, and patients will experience pain with movement of their arms or legs (symptoms of *claudication*). The pain is due to ischemia of the limbs because as the arteries become narrower, circulation becomes more limited. The patient will usually say that the pain stops once the limbs are rested.

### Physical exam in Takayasu's arteritis

On exam, the provider may notice a difference in the blood pressure from one arm to the other. In fact, this is how many patients are first diagnosed. Another name for Takayasu's arteritis is the "*pulseless disease*," as one or more extremities may not have a palpable pulse.

### Diagnosis of Takayasu's arteritis

Diagnosing Takayasu's arteritis can be difficult considering the large vessels cannot be safely biopsied. The most common way to diagnose it is through imaging, the standard being angiography. Angiography visualizes the blood vessel anatomy and evaluates for areas of stenosis **(Fig. 13-3)** or beading (alternating areas of narrowing and aneurysms). In most active cases, the patient has symptoms of systemic involvement such as fatigue, weight loss, fevers, and elevated inflammatory markers (although inflammatory markers are not as consistently elevated as they are in Giant Cell Arteritis).

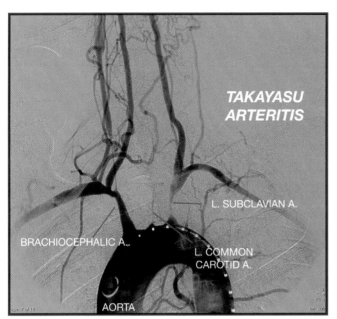

*Figure 13-3.* *Arteriography of the arch of the aorta and main branches in a patient with Takayasu arteritis. Notice the loss of flow in the left common carotid and the left subclavian artery. (A = artery)*

### Treatment of Takayasu's arteritis

No conclusive data exists at this time that shows treatment with any medications are effective besides glucocorticoids. Case series show various immunosuppressive medications are effective, but no large randomized controlled trials have been done to guide therapy. Patients with Takayasu's arteritis are usually treated with a combination of glucocorticoids and DMARD therapy. If DMARD therapy is unsuccessful, then anti-TNF therapy is usually pursued.

# Medium Vessel Vasculitis

## *Polyarteritis Nodosa (PAN)*

*Polyarteritis Nodosa (PAN)* is a medium vessel vasculitis of adults that classically involves the mesenteric blood vessels (blood vessels to the intestines). The name comes from *poly* (many), *arteritis* (inflamed arteries), and *nodosa* (knot-like) because the arteries were described as a rope with many knots in it from multiple aneurysms. For unknown reasons, PAN is highly associated with hepatitis B infections. Since the development of the hepatitis B vaccine, the rate of this diagnosis has decreased greatly.

### History and Physical Exam in PAN

Specific symptoms arise from whatever organs are being involved in PAN.

*Gastrointestinal tract vessel involvement.* The blood vessels to the intestines become inflamed and develop multiple aneurysms, which can develop blood clots and cause downstream ischemia of the blood vessel. The patient complains of weight loss, pain after eating (*mesenteric angina*), and bloody stools from the intestinal ischemia.

*Peripheral nerves.* Narrowing of the medium arteries of the limbs can cause ischemia to peripheral motor and sensory nerves, which can result in sensory and motor loss in the affected limb. A patient may complain of decreasing sensation in a foot, and then gradually or suddenly lose the ability to lift the foot from the ground (*foot drop*).

*Kidneys.* The arteries in the kidney weaken and develop multiple aneurysms. The aneurysms can predispose to thrombus formation within the kidney and cause infarcts. The patient may present with flank pain and hypertension.

*Testicular.* A young patient may develop a testicular pain and a mass that looks like malignancy.

### Diagnosis of PAN

Unfortunately, no diagnostic blood test exists for the diagnosis of PAN. The workup depends on what area of the body the vasculitis is attacking.

*Hepatitis B.* As mentioned before, PAN is associated with hepatitis B; if the diagnosis of PAN is suspected, check hepatitis B serologies.

*Peripheral nerve involvement.* If a patient presents with loss of sensation and motor function in the foot/ankle, then an EMG will classically show a *mononeuritis multiplex*. This refers to both sensory and motor peripheral neuropathy of more than one nerve, which is not specific for vasculitis and can also occur in other conditions. If the EMG is consistent with mononeuritis multiplex, then a biopsy can be taken of a nerve near the affected ankle that only has sensory function (so there is no loss of motor function on removing the nerve); the tissue may reveal vasculitis of the blood vessels around the nerve, which will prove the diagnosis.

*Vascular imaging.* Multiple imaging modalities can image blood vessels, including Computer Tomography Angiography (CTA), Magnetic Resonance Angiography (MRA), and direct angiography, which directly injects contrast into a blood vessel; and x-ray imaging of the injected contrast will reveal the shape of the blood vessel. When imaging of the blood vessels of the intestines (mesenteric arteries) shows evidence of a vasculitis (areas of stenosis and aneurysms) **(Fig. 13-4)**, PAN is a possible cause. Imaging is most helpful in areas that cannot be biopsied, such as the mesenteric vessels. Renal vasculature should also be evaluated when suspecting PAN. A CT of the abdomen can also be helpful, which may show multiple renal infarcts from small thrombi.

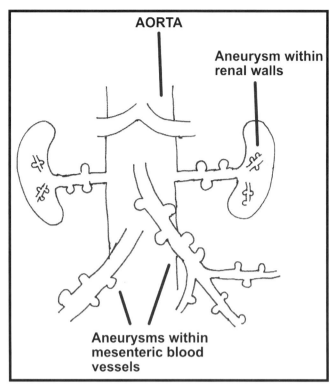

**Figure 13-4.** *Mesenteric and renal blood vessels in a patient with polyarteritis nodosa.*

*Testicular mass.* Biopsy of a testicular mass will reveal vasculitis rather than a malignancy.

### Treatment of PAN

If concomitantly infected with hepatitis B, antivirals should be initiated along with aggressive immunosuppression. Again, no randomized controlled trials exist for the treatment of PAN, and the optimal treatment is unknown. Historically, aggressive therapy with cyclophosphamide is given initially.

## Central Nervous System (CNS) Vasculitis

*CNS vasculitis* is a rare form of vasculitis that usually presents with headaches or ischemic stroke caused by inflammation within the cerebral blood vessels (vasculitis) causing narrowing and decreased blood flow. CNS vasculitis is often suspected when a young patient presents with stroke-like symptoms and brain imaging shows ischemia in multiple areas of the brain. Imaging may show diffuse narrowing of blood vessels within the brain, which raises suspicion for vasculitis. Remember, antiphospholipid syndrome is another cause of stroke in a young patient, but patients with antiphospholipid syndrome should not have narrowing of the blood vessels on imaging.

When CNS vasculitis is suspected, a lumbar puncture should be performed that will demonstrate cerebrospinal fluid with an elevated white blood cell count or elevated protein, which gives a clue to an inflammatory condition in the brain. Infections such as neurosyphilis and herpes zoster can also present with strokes and narrowed cerebral blood vessels and a cerebrospinal fluid with elevated white blood cells and protein, so these infections should be tested for in the patient's serum as well as cerebrospinal fluid. The only way to definitively diagnose CNS vasculitis is a brain biopsy.

## Reversible Cerebral Vasoconstriction Syndrome (RCVS)

*RCVS* is not a vasculitis, but it mimics CNS vasculitis so you should know a little about it. RCVS occurs when the cerebral arteries vasospasm, decreasing blood flow to various areas in the brain. The constriction caused by a vasospasm in RCVS is *not* from inflammation, like you would see in vasculitis; the vasospasm occurs because of an abnormal response to a variety of stimuli, such as high amounts of caffeine, strenuous activity, or exposure to decongestants. It's like Raynaud's phenomenon in the fingers, but in the brain.

RCVS presents as a sudden, severe headache (*thunderclap headache*), commonly described as the worst headache the patient has ever experienced. The headache often occurs during exercise or another form of strenuous activity. Imaging may show blood vessel narrowing, like you see in CNS vasculitis, but the important differentiator is that the cerebrospinal fluid will be normal. The cerebrospinal fluid will not have an elevated white blood cell count or protein because the vasospasm is not caused by inflammation but by an abnormal response to stimuli.

Calcium channel blockers have been used for treatment of RCVS, but patients should be advised to avoid high amounts of caffeine or decongestants.

## Behcet's Disease

Remember ulcers, ulcers, ulcers! This is the disease of oral and genital ulcers. Herpes Simplex Virus is by far a more common cause of oral and genital ulcers, but once herpes has been ruled out (ulcerations are swabbed for virus culture or polymerase chain reaction testing), consider Behcet's disease!

### History and Physical Exam

Behcet's is a unique vasculitis in that it mostly occurs in patients of "silk road" or Mediterranean ancestry (Turkey, Greece, and Israel). It presents very differently from the other systemic vasculitides in that nearly every patient's chief complaint will be *oral* and *genital ulcers*.

*Oral ulcers.* Oral ulcers are usually the first sign of the disease, whether a single ulcer or a crop of many that can last up to 2 weeks, usually healing without scarring. They can occur anywhere in the mouth and are usually very painful.

*Genital ulcers.* Genital ulcers occur slightly less often than oral ulcers but look similar, usually a little larger. The genital ulcers scar more often than the oral ulcers, leaving a hypopigmented area. In males, scrotal lesions are much more common than penile lesions. Females usually have the lesions in the vulvar, vaginal, and cervical areas.

Other signs and symptoms of Behcet's include:

*Ocular disease.* Eye involvement (inflammation in the anterior or posterior aspect of the eye, *anterior* or *posterior uveitis*) is frequent in Behcet's and can cause blindness in 25% of patients if untreated.

*Lungs.* One of the unique aspects of Behcet's is that it is practically the only vasculitis that can involve the *medium-sized* pulmonary arteries and cause pulmonary artery aneurysms. Polyarteritis nodosa, which is a classic medium-sized vasculitis, does not involve the pulmonary arteries for unknown reasons.

*Blood clots.* A major morbidity of patients with Behcet's is *venous* and *arterial thrombosis*. Behcet's is one of the rare instances where thrombosis is treated with aggressive immunosuppression as well as anticoagulation.

### Diagnosis of Behcet's disease

Unfortunately, there isn't a blood test for Behcet's, but one thing you can ask to help clarify the diagnosis is whether the patient has experienced *pathergy*. Pathergy is a skin reaction some patients with Behcet's experience after any sort of trauma or break in the skin. The body reacts more violently to a break in the skin (from a needle stick, for example), and a raised red lesion will develop. If the patient confirms this, it could be pathergy, giving you a clue to the diagnosis.

Oral ulcers that are herpes negative do not mean the patient has Behcet's disease. Oral ulcers of unclear etiology are fairly common in the general population. In order to diagnose Behcet's, the patient should have other aspects of the disease, such as eye involvement, venous/arterial blood clots, and a history of pathergy.

### Treatment of Behcet's disease

Like most diseases in rheumatology, the treatment of Behcet's depends on its severity. If the disease is mild with occasional oral sores, these can be treated with topical or oral glucocorticoids and colchicine. *Apremilast* has been shown effective in treating the ulcers.

In more severe disease, more aggressive immunosuppression is required with DMARD therapy, tumor necrosis factor inhibitors, or cyclophosphamide.

# ANCA-Associated Vasculitis (Small Blood Vessels)

*ANCA-associated vasculitis* is small vessel vasculitis with a positive serum ANCA (Anti-Neutrophilic Cytoplasmic Antibody). ANCA vasculitis is comprised of 3 rare diseases: *Granulomatosis with Polyangiitis, Microscopic Polyangiitis,* and *Eosinophilic Granulomatosis with Polyangiitis.* These 3 diseases all have small vessel involvement, pulmonary involvement, as well as blood test positivity for ANCA. The presentations for these diseases are similar but there are a few keys differences **(Fig. 13-5)**.

## Granulomatosis with Polyangiitis (GPA; Wegener's Disease)

*Granulomatosis with Polyangiitis (GPA)*, formerly called *Wegener's Disease*, is a vasculitis that affects many different blood vessels throughout the body, most commonly in the sinuses, lungs, and kidneys. This type of vasculitis

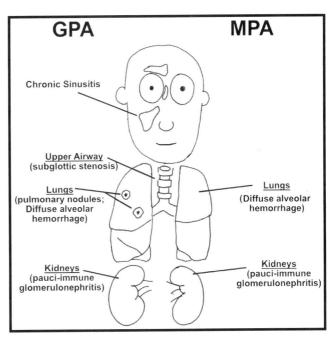

*Figure 13-5. Differences between clinical manifestations of microscopic polyangiitis (MPA) and granulomatosis with polyangiitis (GPA).*

can have necrotizing granulomas on biopsy of affected tissue; hence the "granulomatosis" in the name. Suspect this disease whenever someone has unexplained renal failure and any sort of lung abnormality, like a pneumonia that doesn't improve with antibiotics. GPA can involve the kidneys alone, or just the sinuses and ears, so you shouldn't discard the diagnosis just because only one organ is involved.

## History and Physical Exam of GPA

*Sinuses/ENT. Sinuses are more often the initial area involved in GPA.* Classically, the patient complains of sinus congestion with no relief from over-the-counter antihistamines or nasal sprays. There may be crusting in the nose and bleeding as well. The nasal inflammation can be severe enough to cause a perforation within the nose (septal perforation) or a collapse of structure (*saddle nose deformity*) **(Fig. 13-6)**. Ears can also be involved, with hearing loss or a sense of fullness in the ear. Look into the nose of a patient suspected of having GPA, and evaluate for bleeding, septal perforation, or ulcerations.

*Lung involvement.* The pulmonary presentation in GPA can vary greatly. It can be an asymptomatic

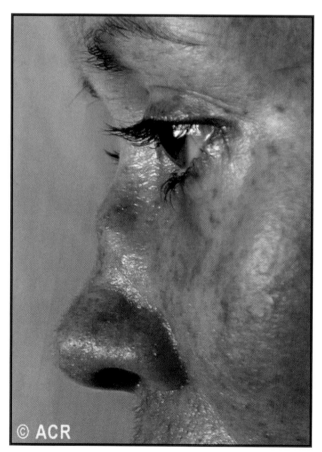

*Figure 13-6. Saddle nose deformity. Image courtesy of the American College of Rheumatology.*

granulomatous nodule or a life-threatening bleeding in the lungs (*diffuse alveolar hemorrhage*).

Diffuse alveolar hemorrhage occurs because of severe inflammation within the small pulmonary vessels/ capillaries, presenting as acute respiratory failure along with coughing up blood (*hemoptysis*). The hemorrhage arises from the smallest blood vessels, the pulmonary capillaries, which "leak" from inflammation within the vessel (vasculitis). X-ray of the chest shows a diffuse fluffy pattern of infiltrate. Hemoglobin may decrease, giving a clue to the cause of hypoxia. Patients with diffuse alveolar hemorrhage usually end up intubated in the ICU. The only way to diagnose it with certainty is by bronchoscopy, which reveals severe bleeding within the airways.

GPA can also present as pulmonary masses or even cavitary lesions. These can be difficult to distinguish from an infection or malignancy. It is important that these patients are seen by a pulmonologist, who can do a bronchoscopy and biopsy to help better determine the cause.

*Kidney involvement.* GPA causes a *glomerulonephritis*, an inflammation in the kidneys caused by the vasculitis. The creatinine will be elevated, and there will be blood in the urine. If you collect the urine, centrifuge it and evaluate it under a microscope; you should be able to see "active sediment," which means *red blood cell casts*. These are tubular aggregates of red blood cells that formed in the kidney tubules during inflammation. If RBC casts are seen, you have a good chance of making your tissue diagnosis with a renal biopsy. Red blood cell casts will not be recognized by sending the urine for a laboratory evaluation because the casts only last a few minutes to hours before dissolving. To detect casts, the urine must be looked at within a few minutes of giving the sample.

A kidney biopsy in active GPA will classically show a *pauci-immune* glomerulonephritis. *Pauci-immune* means very few immune deposits, such as antibodies and complement, which are routinely stained by the pathologist. These deposits are always checked because they are positive in autoimmune diseases like systemic lupus erythematosus. In ANCA-associated vasculitis, however, there is minimal deposition of complement or immunoglobulin. If a patient has pauci-immune glomerulonephritis in the right clinical scenario (diffuse alveolar hemorrhage, sinusitis, positive ANCA), the diagnosis of GPA can be made more confidently.

*Eyes and ears.* Other areas that can be involved are the eyes and ears. Patients can present with swelling around the eyes, sometimes even to the point where they can't open them. The swelling can come and go or it can persist.

*Skin lesions.* GPA can involve the skin, causing erythematous lesions that are palpable to touch referred to as *palpable purpura*. *Purpura* specifically refers to lesions that are non-blanching on exam. *Non-blanching* means that when the examiner pushes into the lesion, the lesion does not briefly turn white (*blanching*). *Palpable* means the lesions are raised from the skin and can be appreciated on exam by running your finger over the skin. Palpable purpura forms when small hemorrhages form under the skin from vascular inflammation.

*Lab testing in GPA* is often positive for **C-ANCA** antibody against **PR3** protein.

## Microscopic Polyangiitis (MPA)

*Microscopic Polyangiitis (MPA)* resembles GPA in that it is a small vessel systemic vasculitis that affects the kidneys and the lungs, but it is not associated with granulomas on biopsy. The patient will *NOT have* the additional complications of sinus and hearing problems you may find in GPA.

MPA often presents with kidney failure and glomerulonephritis, and the renal biopsy will look identical to that in GPA. The lung involvement of MPA is diffuse alveolar hemorrhage; MPA does not cause pulmonary nodules as seen in GPA.

*Lab testing in MPA* is often positive for P-ANCA antibody against MPO protein.

### Diagnosis of GPA and MPA

Diagnosis is made with a combination of symptoms, lab findings (ANCA positivity), and tissue biopsy when possible.

### Treatment of GPA and MPA

Treatment of GPA and MPA depends on the severity of disease and can be divided into organ-threatening and non-organ-threatening disease.

*Non-organ-threatening disease.* An example would be a patient with sinusitis, joint pains, and scattered pulmonary nodules that are found to be C-ANCA/PR3 positive with pulmonary nodule biopsy, demonstrating necrotizing granuloma and vasculitis. This patient could be treated with glucocorticoids in combination with the steroid-sparing agent, methotrexate.

*Organ-threatening disease.* An example would be a patient presenting with hypoxia, coughing up blood, as well as an elevated creatinine, kidney biopsy showing pauci-immune glomerulonephritis, and bronchoscopy revealing diffuse alveolar hemorrhage. This patient has life-threatening disease and requires high-dose glucocorticoids as well as induction therapy with either rituximab or cyclophosphamide.

## Goodpasture's Disease

*Goodpasture's disease* presents similarly to MPA and GPA, namely bleeding in the lungs as well as glomerulonephritis. The difference is that the kidney biopsy shows antibody deposits in the kidney, classically in a linear staining pattern (not pauci-immune), and the patient will also have anti-GBM (Glomerular Basement Membrane) antibodies in the blood.

## Eosinophilic Granulomatosis with Polyangiitis (EGPA; Churg-Strauss)

Think of this disease when you see adult onset asthma and eosinophilia! EGPA, previously called *Churg-Strauss Syndrome,* is considered in the category of ANCA vasculitis, but confusingly only half of patients will have a positive ANCA (P-ANCA, MPO), which can make the diagnosis a little more difficult. It is considered ANCA-associated because half of patients will have a positive ANCA titer, but in other vasculitides like GPA, the ANCA positivity is much more prevalent.

Two important characteristics of EGPA help separate it from GPA and MPA:

- *Eosinophilia.* The most striking characteristic of EGPA is the associated eosinophilia (usually >10%).
- *Asthma.* The initial symptom is usually difficult-to-treat asthma that develops months to years prior to other symptoms.

Other complaints include:

- *Sinus symptoms.* Chronic congestion
- *Lung involvement.* Patients may develop shortness of breath, but EGPA is less likely to have diffuse alveolar hemorrhage compared to GPA or MPA.

Remember EGPA in a patient with adult onset asthma and eosinophilia!

Two other important characteristics of EGPA are:

- *Foot or wrist drop.* Initially this usually occurs unilaterally, most often in the foot/ankle. The patient notices a loss of sensation in the foot and then within days to weeks will no longer be able to dorsiflex the ankle. The combination of sensory and motor loss is consistent with a *mononeuritis multiplex*, described above with polyarteritis nodosa.
- *Cardiomyopathy.* EGPA has an unfortunate tendency to involve cardiac tissue and cause a severe cardiomyopathy, which can be fatal if untreated. A patient with EGPA presenting with symptoms suggestive of heart failure needs a cardiac MRI, which will show cardiac inflammation within the cardiac muscle.

### Diagnosis of EGPA

The diagnosis of EGPA can be difficult because multiple systems may be involved and asthma may present years before additional clinical manifestations appear. The American College of Rheumatology diagnostic criteria are as follows:

If a patient has 4 or more of the following 6 findings, the specificity of an EGPA diagnosis is 99%:

- asthma
- > 10% eosinophils in the serum
- neurologic involvement, such as foot drop
- *transient and migratory pulmonary opacities.* (These findings take weeks to months to produce as a patient needs to have chest x-rays multiple times showing an opacity in one area of the lung, then resolution of the initial opacity, and an opacity in another area, referred to as *migratory opacity.*)
- paranasal sinus abnormality-congestion, crusting in the nose, nosebleed
- biopsy of skin/lung/nerve demonstrating accumulation of eosinophils and vasculitis

### Treatment of EGPA

Like most diseases in rheumatology, the treatment of EGPA depends on the severity of disease. Glucocorticoids rapidly reduce eosinophils and can be used acutely, but steroid-sparing agents are required for long-term management. Long-term management options include cyclophosphamide, rituximab, methotrexate, and azathioprine. The newer promising agent *mepolizumab* targets and blocks interleukin-5, which has been shown to drive eosinophil production and is less toxic than cyclophosphamide.

### ANCA lab testing

The 2 antibodies in ANCA vasculitis are *Cytoplasmic (C-ANCA)* and *Peri-nuclear (P-ANCA)*. These tests are done as a first step by immunofluorescence, which requires a pathologist to microscopically examine cells and evaluate if the immunofluorescence is consistent with a cytoplasmic pattern (C-ANCA) or a perinuclear pattern (P-ANCA). If the pathologist detects either a C-ANCA or a P-ANCA pattern, then an *ELISA test* (Enzyme Linked Immunosorbent Assay) will be performed. This test looks for the protein that the C- or P-ANCA is targeting. The two most common proteins are *MPO* and *PR3*. C-ANCA usually coincides with PR3, while P-ANCA usually coincides with MPO. Ideally, a patient will have ANCA positivity as well as either the PR3 or the MPO **(Fig. 13-7)**. If these tests are positive, this increases the specificity of the diagnosis considerably. Occasionally a patient will be P-ANCA positive, but negative for both PR3 and MPO, which is much less specific for the diagnosis of ANCA vasculitis.

## ANCA Not Associated With Vasculitis

It is important to understand that a positive ANCA does not mean a patient has vasculitis. Much like a positive ANA, ANCA needs to be looked at in the appropriate clinical context. The following are examples of drugs/medications and infections that can cause a positive ANCA lab test and may not have a corresponding vasculitis.

*Medication-induced ANCA.* Certain medications, e.g. hydralazine and propothiouracil, can cause a positive ANCA test. A clue that the positive ANCA is drug-induced may be dual positivity of the ANCA. This means that both C- and P-ANCA are positive with corresponding PR3 and MPO positivity. Usually GPA, MPA or EGPA will have either C-ANCA and PR3 or P-ANCA and MPO, not both. When both are present, consider medication-induced vasculitis.

*Drug-induced ANCA.* The drug most associated with ANCA vasculitis is cocaine. Cocaine itself likely does not cause the vasculitis, but *levamisole*, a common cocaine adulterant, can. The presentation of cocaine-induced vasculitis is necrotic-appearing skin, usually around the patient's ears, cheeks, and nose. It is usually a cutaneous-limited vasculitis that may or may not have a positive ANCA blood test. If the patient has necrotic-appearing skin on different areas of the face as well as a positive urine cocaine toxicology screen, this should be enough for the diagnosis.

| FIGURE 13-7.  LABS & ORGAN INVOLVEMENT IN ANCA-ASSOCIATED VASCULITIDES | | |
|---|---|---|
| **ANCA Vasculitis** | **ANCA** | **Major Organs Involved** |
| Wegener's (GPA) | 90% C-ANCA, PR3 | Sinus, Lung, Kidney |
| Microscopic Polyangiitis (MPA) | 80% P-ANCA, MPO | Lung, Kidney |
| Eosinophilic Granulomatosis with Polyangiitis (EGPA) | 50% P-ANCA, MPO | Sinus, Lung, Nerves |

**Infection-induced ANCA.** The most serious infectious cause of a positive ANCA is bacterial endocarditis, which can look a lot like GPA. A patient with infectious endocarditis may have pulmonary nodules, glomerulonephritis, and a variety of skin lesions, including palpable purpura.

Other primary diseases can also have a positive ANCA, most commonly *inflammatory bowel disease* and *cystic fibrosis*.

## Cryoglobulinemic Vasculitis

*Cryoglobulinemic vasculitis* is also a small/medium vessel vasculitis, but it is not associated with ANCA positivity. Before we discuss cryoglobulinemic vasculitis, it's important to define *cryoglobulins*.

- Cryoglobulins are antibodies in the blood that are no longer soluble in the blood (precipitate out of the blood) below 37°C, but then dissolve again upon rewarming to 37°C.
- Cryoglobulinemia is the presence of cryoglobulins within blood.

Healthy individuals have very low levels of cryoglobulins, but increased levels are associated with hepatitis C as well as hematologic conditions that produce increased antibodies, such as multiple myeloma; Waldenstrom macroglobulinemia; monoclonal gammopathy of undetermined significance; and autoimmune diseases that produce increased amount of antibodies, such as systemic lupus erythematosus and Sjögren's syndrome.

Multiple types of cryoglobulinemia exist; the type depends on the underlying disease process, e.g. hepatitis C or multiple myeloma. Cryoglobulinemic vasculitis occurs when the cryoglobulins precipitate out of the blood, triggering an inflammatory cascade within the blood vessels, hence a vasculitis. Cryoglobulinemic vasculitis can affect a variety of organ systems, similar to other small/medium vessel vasculitities. Other signs include:

- joint pains
- palpable skin purpura similar to that seen in ANCA vasculitis as well as distal skin ulcerations
- Renal biopsy shows a membranoproliferative glomerulonephritis that displays evidence of thrombi in the tissue positive for IgM and IgG. This differs from ANCA vasculitis, which can show a glomerulonephritis without IgM or IgG staining (*pauci-immune*).
- sensory and motor loss in a foot or hand, similar to that seen in ANCA vasculitis

## Diagnosis of cryoglobulinemic vasculitis

Laboratory testing is critical in the evaluation of cryoglobulinemic vasculitis. The presence of cryoglobulins can be tested in the blood by cooling the serum and evaluating for precipitation of protein, which over days appears like sand at the bottom of a cooled tube of serum. Once cryoglobulins are detected, the specific types of antibodies can then be evaluated, which will give a clue to the cause of the cryoglobulins, such as chronic infection vs hematologic disease vs autoimmune disease. Hepatitis C is by far the most common cause of cryoglobulinemic vasculitis.

Testing for cryoglobulins in the blood can take multiple days and needs to be done in a laboratory equipped for the testing.

## Treatment of cryoglobulinemic vasculitis

Treatment depends on the severity of disease as well as what is causing the cryoglobulins, infection vs hematologic process vs autoimmune disease. If hepatitis C is the cause, then treatment of the underlying hepatitis C may cure the vasculitis, but if the patient has severe, organ-threatening disease, aggressive immunosuppression is warranted along with treatment of the underlying cause.

# Cases

1. HISTORY: A 65-year-old man with a history of high cholesterol presents with a 3 month history of severe sinusitis as well as joint pain and swelling that seems to move around. For a few days his left elbow was swollen and painful; then this resolved and his right elbow became painful and swollen. He denies any rashes or changes in urination.
   PHYSICAL EXAM: On exam, nasal crusting is noticed along with an ulcer in his nasal septum. He has limited range of motion of his right elbow with mild warmth and minimal effusion appreciated.
   LABORATORY: During the workup, he is found to have a positive C-ANCA, PR3. His chest x-ray and kidney function are normal, with no blood in the urine.
   DIAGNOSIS: Granulomatosis with Polyangiitis (GPA)
   TREATMENT: This patient can be initiated on prednisone to quickly help his joint pain and sinus congestion. He has clinical features consistent with non-organ-threatening GPA (no lung, nerve, or renal involvement). He can be treated less aggressively with weekly methotrexate, and watched closely.

**2.** HISTORY: 54-year-old woman presents with a 1 month history of weight loss, fatigue, recent development of shortness of breath, and coughing up small amounts of blood. She was treated in the past week for pneumonia with antibiotics, but her symptoms do not seem to be improving.

PHYSICAL EXAM: Respiratory rate of 30, oxygen saturation of 84% on room air. She appears uncomfortable. Her pulmonary exam is notable for diffuse rales in all lung fields. She also has palpable purpura in her lower extremities bilaterally.

LABS AND IMAGING: Her chest imaging reveals diffuse alveolar infiltrate; her hemoglobin is low at 7g/dl; and her creatinine is 4.6mg/dl along with blood in her urine. Red blood cell casts are appreciated on urine microscopy. C-ANCA positive and PR3 positive.

DIAGNOSIS: This patient likely has organ- and life-threatening GPA.

TREATMENT: She needs to be hospitalized in the intensive care unit and monitored closely. Considering the presence of red blood cell casts, a renal biopsy can be pursued for a more definitive diagnosis. For treatment, she will require high-dose intravenous glucocorticoids as well as either cyclosphosphamide or rituximab.

# 14

# Inflammatory Myopathies

An *inflammatory myopathy* is an autoimmune disease that destroys muscle cells by inflammatory cells such as lymphocytes and macrophages infiltrating muscle tissue. *Non-inflammatory myopathy* is a more general term used to describe dysfunction of a muscle that isn't secondary to inflammation, e.g. muscular dystrophy. Inflammatory myopathies differ from most other rheumatologic diseases in that they do not involve the joints (usually). In patients with inflammatory myopathies, the immune system attacks and destroys the patient's muscles, not the joints, so these patients do not have synovitis; they have weakness.

In this chapter, inflammatory myopathy refers to *polymyositis*, *dermatomyositis*, and *necrotizing myopathy*, the three major idiopathic inflammatory myopathies. *Inclusion body myositis (IBM)* is also considered an inflammatory myopathy, but we will discuss this disease separately, as it presents differently and has a different prognosis.

## History in Inflammatory Myopathy

*Proximal muscle weakness.* The weakness that occurs in inflammatory myopathy is unique. It affects the proximal muscle groups and spares the distal muscle groups (hands and feet). Patients may complain specifically of weakness in the muscles of the shoulder and thighs. The patient will not be able to hold up the arms for long periods of time, as in combing the hair, without the arms feeling exhausted. The patient will also describe difficulty standing from a seated position, such as getting up off the toilet. Classically, the patient will not have any weakness in hand grip or plantar-dorsiflexion of the foot (distal muscles).

*Painless weakness.* Pain is only rarely associated with inflammatory myopathies. The patient can't hold up the arms because of loss of strength, not because of pain.

*No sensory loss.* Patients with inflammatory myopathies should have normal sensation throughout the body. If the patient complains of loss of sensation in the extremities, think of another diagnosis.

The *diaphragm* and *esophagus* may also be involved. If a patient describes difficulty breathing or swallowing, take this seriously. If untreated, respiratory arrest can follow.

Weakness is a very common complaint in a general practitioner's office. Ascertain whether the weakness is generalized (deconditioning from lack of exercise or from anemia) or more specific, which could be either neurologic (Guillain-Barré, multiple sclerosis, amyotrophic lateral sclerosis) or muscular (inherited myopathies, muscular dystrophy, or inflammatory myopathy). Causes of weakness are numerous, but make sure you can recognize the pattern of painless, proximal muscle weakness that is seen in the inflammatory myopathies.

## Polymyositis, Dermatomyositis And Necrotizing Myopathy

*Polymyositis (PM)*, *dermatomyositis (DM)*, and *necrotizing myopathy* are the most important idiopathic inflammatory myopathies to know about. Skin manifestations are seen in dermatomyositis (hence the "derm" in the name), while polymyositis and necrotizing myopathy do not have skin changes. There are also differences in their muscle biopsy results that can help differentiate the diseases if the skin manifestations are not obvious. The treatment of all three is similar.

Dermatomyositis has an association with underlying malignancy. Patients recently diagnosed with dermatomyositis should undergo age-appropriate cancer screening or more advanced screening, depending on symptoms (e.g. chest imaging in the setting of cough).

## Physical Exam

### Upper Extremity Weakness

*Proximal.* Ask the patient to raise the arms above the head and resist your pulling down on the arms. *Distal.* Ask the patient to grip and squeeze your fingers, as well as spread the fingers and resist your attempt to push the fingers together; then resist your flexing or extending the fingers.

### Lower Extremity Weakness

*Proximal.* While the patient is lying down, ask the patient to raise one leg off the table as high as possible, then push down on the thigh and see if the patient can resist the downward force. *Distal.* Ask the patient to dorsiflex or plantar flex the feet against resistance.

### Skin involvement

This is the first aspect of the patient workup that will differentiate the inflammatory myopathies. Patients with dermatomyositis (DM) complain of skin changes that gradually accompany the muscle weakness. The rashes are often photosensitive, meaning they worsen when exposed to sunlight. Patients may present with any one or a combination of the following:

**Note:** *The patient just needs one of the following skin findings to increase suspicion of DM.*

- *Heliotrope rash:* a red/purple rash on the eyelids and around the eyes **(Fig. 14-1)**
- *Shawl sign:* an erythematous rash that develops on the upper chest and wraps around to the upper back
- *Gottron's papules:* an erythematous raised rash on the extensor surfaces of the finger joints **(Fig. 14-2)**
- *Holster sign:* an erythematous lesion on the lateral aspect of the upper thigh; it looks like the patient is wearing a holster for a gun.

## Diagnosis of Inflammatory Myopathy

### Labs

The most important laboratory value when evaluating for an inflammatory myopathy is the creatine

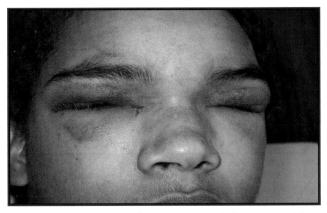

**Figure 14-1.** *Heliotrope rash in a patient with dermatomyositis.*

kinase (CK). In almost all cases of active polymyositis, dermatomyositis, and necrotizing myopathy, the CK will be very elevated, indicating active destruction of muscle cells. The liver enzymes (aspartate aminotransferase and alanine aminotransferase) can also be elevated; this is not due to liver damage but leakage of these enzymes from damaged muscle cells. The patient's white blood cells, erythrocyte sedimentation rate, and C-reactive protein may also be elevated.

Also measure thyroid-stimulating hormone (TSH) and free T4 to make sure the muscle disease is not related to underlying hypothyroidism.

*Antibodies.* Every year new antibodies are discovered that are associated with inflammatory myopathies. One of the more important antibodies to check for is *anti-3-hydroxy-3-methylglutaryl-coenzyme A reductase (HMG-COA reductase).* This antibody is seen in statin-induced necrotizing inflammatory myopathy. Statins are commonly prescribed to lower cholesterol and are associated with muscle cramps and occasional *rhabdomyolysis* (destruction of striated muscle cells). Less commonly, patients on statins can develop an inflammatory myopathy that presents just like the other inflammatory myopathies. On biopsy, the pathology will be consistent with a necrotizing myopathy (see muscle biopsy below). The only way to diagnose HMG-COA reductase myopathy with certainty is by checking the anti-HMG-COA reductase antibody. Statin therapy needs to be stopped, but the patient will also require high-dose immunosuppression therapy. Note that the chemical in statins can be found in certain foods (e.g. mushrooms and rice), so a patient does not have to be on a statin to develop this disease.

### Procedures and Imaging

An *electromyogram (EMG)* is crucial in the workup of inflammatory myopathy because it can help distinguish if the weakness originates from the nerves or the

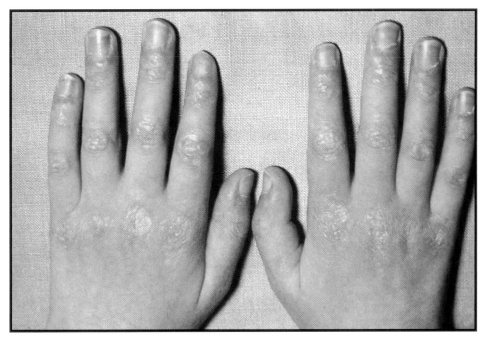

*Figure 14-2.* Gottron's papules. Erythematous raised lesions on the dorsum of the joints of the fingers. Image courtesy of the American College of Rheumatology.

muscle. The muscle will be the source of abnormalities seen in inflammatory myopathy, whereas the nerves will be abnormal in diseases that damage the nerves, such as forms of vasculitis. The EMG can also show areas of abnormality that are a high-yield place for muscle biopsy. (Biopsy should be done on the opposite leg of the EMG in the same location, since the EMG can actually cause muscle changes, which will confuse the biopsy results).

*MRI* is the most important imaging technique when working up a patient for inflammatory myopathy, but it is not always necessary. MRI can demonstrate areas of muscle inflammation, edema, and necrosis. The imaging results are not diagnostic of inflammatory myopathy, so the imaging findings can be used to guide a muscle biopsy to an area of active inflammation.

### Muscle Biopsy

The combination of proximal muscle weakness and skin changes (in dermatomyositis) with the corresponding muscle biopsy results can establish the diagnosis of inflammatory myopathy.

*Polymyositis:* Lymphocytes appear *around and within* the muscle cells (compare **Figs. 14-3, 14-4**).

*Dermatomyositis.* Lymphocytes infiltrating *around* the muscle cell along with *perifascicular atrophy* (compare **Figs. 14-3, 14-5**). Perifascicular atrophy is atrophy of the muscle cells at the periphery of the muscle fascicles. The muscle cells farther away from the fascicle are not atrophied. Blood vessels around the muscle may show

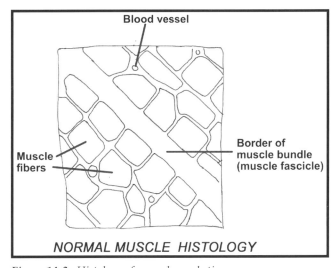

*Figure 14-3.* Histology of normal muscle tissue.

inflammation as well in dermatomyositis.

*Necrotizing myopathy* manifests as necrosis of muscle cells. Importantly, macrophages infiltrate the muscle cells rather than lymphocytes.

## *Other Causes of Muscle Weakness*

The differential diagnosis for weakness is very broad, so it's critical to get a good history on patients presenting with weakness. Here are a few less common diseases that present with weakness and need to be excluded when diagnosing an inflammatory myopathy.

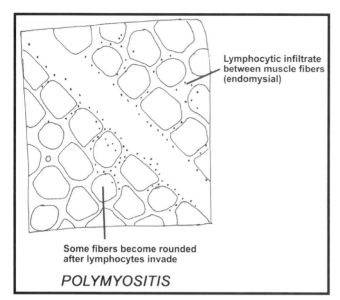

Lymphocytic infiltrate between muscle fibers (endomysial)

Some fibers become rounded after lymphocytes invade

**POLYMYOSITIS**

*Figure 14-4.* Muscle histology of polymyositis, showing lymphocytic infiltrate between and within the muscle cells.

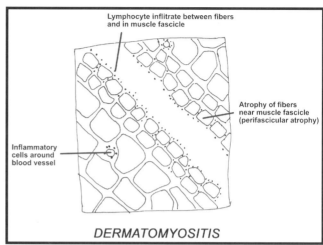

Lymphocyte infiltrate between fibers and in muscle fascicle

Atrophy of fibers near muscle fascicle (perifascicular atrophy)

Inflammatory cells around blood vessel

**DERMATOMYOSITIS**

*Figure 14-5.* Muscle histology of dermatomyositis. Notice the atrophy of the muscle cells near the fascicle as well as inflammation around the blood vessels (perivascular infiltrate).

## Muscular Dystrophies

*Muscular dystrophies* are a group of muscle disorders caused by abnormal gene mutations that change the production of proteins needed for healthy muscle. Muscular dystrophies contrast with inflammatory myopathies, where the primary driver of the disease is autoimmunity and inflammation with destruction of the muscle. There are many different muscular dystrophies, and new ones are being discovered each year. It's a bit overwhelming to approach a patient with weakness and attempt to rule out muscular dystrophy as a cause, but here are a few things to keep in mind:

- Muscular dystrophies are *inherited* diseases and often present in adolescents and young adults.
- Often the patients will have additional muscle involvement besides the proximal muscles seen in inflammatory myopathies, such as the facial muscles or scapular winging.
- Different types of stains can be done on a muscle biopsy, which will give clues to protein abnormalities in the diagnosis of muscular dystrophies. The muscle biopsy, while important for the diagnosis of inflammatory myopathy, can also help exclude other causes such as muscular dystrophies.

## Metabolic Myopathies

*Metabolic myopathies* are a group of hereditary muscle disorders (e.g. glycogen storage diseases) caused by a defect in certain enzymes needed for normal muscle function. There are many types of metabolic myopathies, A few points will help direct you toward them:

- *Exercise.* Exercise may make the weakness of a metabolic myopathy much worse. The patient may feel normal without exercise, but weak on starting to exercise. This contrasts with inflammatory myopathy, which is weak at baseline regardless of activity level.
- *Fasting.* Fasting may trigger the weakness in certain metabolic myopathies. In inflammatory myopathy, eating will not make a major difference.
- *Recent illness.* A recent illness can worsen symptoms of weakness in metabolic myopathies. The patient may be feeling normal, but an upper respiratory tract infection may trigger the weakness, which will resolve within a few days of recovery from the infection.
- *Diagnostic muscle biopsy and gene testing.* Muscle biopsy may reveal characteristic findings of metabolic myopathies. Also, some of the metabolic myopathies can undergo genetic testing.

## Primary Neurologic Diseases

As you can imagine, many neurologic conditions may present with weakness as a complaint. Weakness in neurologic disease occurs when nerves inadequately signal the muscles. The primary derangement is in the nerve and not the muscle. In many neurologic disorders, there is also a component of sensory dysfunction that may help guide the diagnosis, as in Guillain-Barré syndrome and multiple sclerosis. Amyotrophic lateral sclerosis (ALS) does not have a sensory loss component, but other clues to the diagnosis can be gathered, such as

- Proximal AND distal weakness of the upper and lower extremities
- Atrophy, fasciculation, and hyperreflexia (pathognomonic of ALS)

- Speech difficulty, drooling
- Poor coordination

## *Treatment of Inflammatory Myopathy*

The most important treatment for inflammatory myopathy is high doses of glucocorticoids for months. Steroid-sparing agents such as methotrexate and azathioprine are also conventionally used. If the patient has breathing (diaphragmatic) or swallowing difficulty, the patient should be hospitalized immediately and treated with high-dose intravenous steroids and intravenous immunoglobulin (IVIG).

# Inclusion Body Myositis

*Inclusion body myositis (IBM)* is considered an inflammatory myopathy, but it differs from dermatomyositis, polymyositis, and necrotizing myopathy in many significant ways.

*Age.* Patients with IBM are exclusively over 50 years old and usually above 70, compared with the other inflammatory myopathies, which can be seen in the younger population.

*Onset.* The onset of IBM is insidious (it progresses very slowly) and is usually ongoing for 5 years before a diagnosis is made.

*Muscle involvement.* IBM involves distal as well as proximal muscles, and it can often present asymmetrically. If a patient has flexion weakness of the fingers as well as proximal muscles, possibly worse on one arm than another, then consider IBM in the diagnosis.

*Labs.* Typically, the CK is mildly elevated in IBM, but much lower compared to the other inflammatory myopathies.

*Biopsy.* A few things to look for in IBM:

- *Rimmed vacuoles*: focal areas of destruction (like small cut out holes) in the muscle cell
- *Inclusion bodies*: small groups of tubules of filamentous material found in muscle cells on electron microscopy

*Prognosis.* IBM is an important diagnosis to consider, as it does not respond to high-dose immunosuppressants, in contrast with the other inflammatory myopathies. In fact, the diagnosis is often made when a patient is suspected of having polymyositis but does not respond to high-dose glucocorticoids. At this point there is no effective medication for IBM; it is a slowly progressive irreversible disease.

## Malignancy Screening

There is an association of inflammatory myopathy, especially dermatomyositis, and underlying malignancy.

Whenever an inflammatory myopathy is diagnosed, age-appropriate cancer screening should be performed. If a woman has any complaints of abdominal discomfort in the setting of inflammatory myopathy, transvaginal ultrasound or an abdominal CT should be pursued, evaluating for underlying ovarian cancer.

# Overlap Syndromes that Have Inflammatory Myopathy

## *Mixed Connective Tissue Disease (MCTD)*

*Mixed Connective Tissue Disease (MCTD)* is a lupus overlap syndrome that can present with characteristics of lupus (inflammatory arthritis, photosensitive rash), Raynaud's (fingertips change color in the cold, going from white to blue to red), and inflammatory myositis. All of these patients are anti-RNP positive (see Chapter 5, Systemic Lupus Erythematosus for more details).

## *Antisynthetase Syndrome*

*Antisynthetase syndrome* encompasses an overlap of inflammatory myopathy, interstitial lung disease (inflammation and scarring of the lungs), fever, Raynaud's phenomenon, and skin thickening of the hands that produces cracks in the skin (*mechanic's hands*). The patient does not need to exhibit all of these symptoms to be labeled as having antisynthetase syndrome. Once the antibody is discovered, the specificity is high enough for the patient to be labeled with the disease as long as the patient has at least one of the symptoms. *Anti-Jo-1* is the most commonly found antibody in this overlap syndrome. Treatment consists of glucocorticoids and a steroid-sparing agent such as mycophenolate mofetil.

# Cases

1. HISTORY: A 45-year-old woman presents with progressive weakness in her arms and legs over the course of 3 months. She first noticed it while she was getting up off the toilet and feels it has been progressively getting worse. She also noticed some difficulty combing her hair in the mornings because she felt like her arms would just get too tired, and she would have to bring them back down to her sides. She doesn't have pain, just weakness. She notes a purplish discoloration around her eyes and eyelids and wonders if it could be bruising. Also, she has some red raised lumps on the backs of her fingers that she feels are becoming more noticeable.

PHYSICAL EXAM: The patient cannot hold up her arms above her head against resistance. When lying down, she cannot hold up her legs against resistance either. Her finger, hand, ankle, and foot strength are normal. There is a purplish color around her eyes and eyelids when she closes her eyes.

LABS AND PROCEDURES: Creatinine kinase (CK) level is 16,000 IU/L (normal 60-174 IU/L). EMG is performed on her left upper and lower extremities, and the findings are consistent with an inflammatory myopathy. Biopsy performed on her right quadriceps shows lymphocytic infiltrate and perifascicular atrophy.

DIAGNOSIS AND TREATMENT: The combination of clinical presentation, skin findings, and biopsy are consistent with dermatomyositis. She does not report shortness of breath or swallowing difficulties, so hospital admission and high-dose intravenous steroids aren't necessary at this time. However, many of these patients are often admitted to the hospital just to expedite workup, considering so many components need to be evaluated to make the diagnosis. Oral prednisone 60 mg/day with slow taper in combination with azathioprine or methotrexate is reasonable. The patient will not likely feel better immediately, even if the inflammation is stopped with medications; it takes months to rebuild muscle.

Whenever a patient is diagnosed with dermatomyositis, it is imperative to be up to date with cancer screening, as upwards of 20% of patients with a new diagnosis of dermatomyositis have an underlying malignancy.

2. HISTORY: A 65-year-old man with a history of coronary artery disease presents with a multiple-month history of worsening weakness, fatigue and, more recently, shortness of breath. Over the last few weeks he's progressively had more trouble raising himself from a seated position. Now he's in a wheelchair and can't get out of it without assistance. He's able to move his hands and feet without difficulty. He has difficulty swallowing and feels his food is getting stuck in his throat. He's been on a statin to treat his elevated cholesterol for the past 5 years.

PHYSICAL EXAM: He cannot raise his arms above his head or get up from a seated position. His hand grip is normal bilaterally. He cannot extend his neck against resistance. He cannot flex his hips while seated. He can move his legs horizontally across the seat, but he cannot raise his legs off the seat. He has normal dorsi-plantar flexion of the feet.

LABORATORY AND PROCEDURES: CK is 32,000 IU/L (normal 60-174 IU/L). Chest x-ray shows an elevated diaphragm. Pulmonary function tests suggest diaphragmatic weakness. EMG shows evidence of inflammatory myopathy. Biopsy performed on his quadriceps reveals necrotizing myopathy with macrophage infiltrate. Blood tests reveal a positive anti-HMG-COA antibody.

DIAGNOSIS AND TREATMENT: This patient with anti-HMG-COA reductase antibody-associated necrotizing myopathy is critically ill. It is important to note the diaphragmatic and esophageal involvement of the inflammatory myopathy, which prompt aggressive management and hospitalization. This patient needs to be given high-dose intravenous steroids (I,000 mg of intravenous solumedrol) along with intravenous immunoglobulin therapy. Patients with inflammatory myopathy who present critically ill may take months to recover, as the muscle damage is severe. His statin therapy should also be stopped.

# 15

# *Miscellaneous Rheumatologic Diseases*

Diagnosis in rheumatology often involves pattern recognition. For example, progressive joint pain and swelling in the small joints of the hands (symmetric), worse in the morning and better with activity, is consistent with rheumatoid arthritis. Many diagnoses in rheumatology don't fit into a broad category such as inflammatory arthritis, but are diagnosed by the recognition of certain patterns on presentation. This chapter categorizes autoimmune diseases based on the more common presenting pattern of the disease. Many of the diseases in this chapter are very rare, but others, like sarcoidosis, are more common and should be on the differential of a variety of clinical presentations.

## Infiltrative Autoimmune Diseases

An infiltrative lesion is a mass-like lesion within a tissue or body cavity that raises concern for malignancy or infection, but occasionally autoimmune diseases can be the cause. Most autoimmune diseases do not cause a mass within a body cavity or organ; thus, when an infiltrative lesion is discovered on imaging, this narrows down the differential from a rheumatologic perspective. The following are examples of the immune system causing a mass-like lesion, usually found on imaging, with subsequent diagnosis upon biopsy. The summary of biopsy findings from these autoimmune infiltrative diseases can be seen in **Figure 15-2.**

## *Sarcoidosis*

*Sarcoidosis* is an autoimmune granulomatous disorder of unknown cause, potentially involving any organ in the body but with a predilection for the lungs (lung involvement in 90% of cases). Most cases of sarcoidosis, for unknown reasons, occur in African Americans. Sarcoidosis is one of the famous diseases you hear about in medical school that can mimic every other disease, so it is important to have it on the differential for a variety of presentations. Histologically, the lesions are defined by the presence of noncaseating granulomas, in contrast to *Mycobacterium tuberculosis* and Granulomatosis with Polyangiitis, both of which are characterized by necrotizing (caseating) granulomas. *Caseating* means cheeselike (the center of the granulomas looks like cheese). On microscopy the caseation appears like a formless mass, without distinguishable cells or nuclei of cells. When a granuloma is described as NONcaseating and has negative fungal stains, the first thing on your mind should be sarcoidosis.

Approximately half of the cases of sarcoidosis are discovered incidentally on radiographs while evaluating another symptom. Classically, the chest radiograph shows bilateral enlarged hilar lymph nodes (*hilar lymphadenopathy*) with widening of the mediastinum **(Fig. 15-1)**. The *hila* are the medial aspects of the lung composed of the pulmonary arteries, veins, and lymphatic vessels. The lymphadenopathy is accessible to biopsy with bronchoscopy.

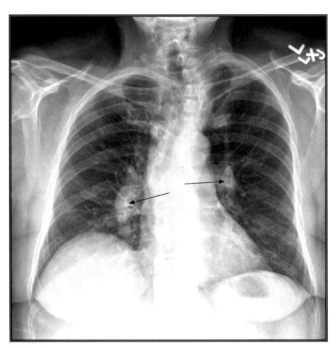

*Figure 15-1. bilateral hilar adenopathy. Notice the prominent masses (arrows) on both sides of the chest in the area of the hilum.*

The presentation of sarcoidosis depends on the organ system(s) involved, although many patients with sarcoidosis are asymptomatic:

*Pulmonary.* The most common presenting symptoms of sarcoidosis are lung-related: cough and shortness of breath, often with fatigue.

*Skin. Cutaneous sarcoidosis* presents with a variety of skin lesions ranging from erythematous plaques to subcutaneous nodules. The diagnosis is often made on biopsy of the lesions, which may reveal noncaseating granulomas. Cutaneous sarcoidosis can manifest in other ways besides granuloma formation; it can also present as *erythema nodosum.*

- Erythema nodosum is a *panniculitis*, meaning inflammation of the subcutaneous adipose tissue. Erythema nodosum presents as tender erythematous nodules, most commonly in the extremities, e.g. the shins. Erythema nodosum is not specific for sarcoidosis; it can be post-infectious or associated with medications (e.g. oral contraceptive pills) or inflammatory bowel disease. Erythema nodosum caused by sarcoidosis is part of a triad called *Löfgren syndrome*, which includes erythema nodosum, hilar lymphadenopathy, and joint pains. Löfgren syndrome is more common in Scandinavian countries as well as Spain.

*Cardiac. Cardiac sarcoidosis* disrupts the cardiac muscles, leading to impaired heart function (heart failure). Suspect cardiac sarcoidosis when a patient has unexplained heart failure along with an MRI showing infiltrative lesions in the heart muscle.

*Lymph nodes.* Lymph node involvement by sarcoidosis causes lymph node enlargement (*lymphadenopathy*), appreciated on physical exam or imaging. It can mimic lymphoma.

*Central Nervous System.* Brain involvement is rare for sarcoidosis, but it is important to include in the differential, since it can mimic a tumor. Symptoms depend on what area of the brain is involved. A clue to the diagnosis is an elevated white blood cell count and elevated protein in the cerebrospinal fluid, along with a mildly low glucose (this can be seen in infectious meningitis as well, so infection needs to be ruled out).

No lab tests are diagnostic of sarcoidosis at the time of this writing. Elevated serum angiotensin-converting enzyme (ACE) levels have been evaluated as a diagnostic tool, but an elevated level is neither sensitive nor specific for the diagnosis.

The treatment of sarcoidosis depends on whether or not it is causing organ damage. If sarcoidosis is found on imaging and biopsy, but is not causing organ damage or symptoms, it is reasonable to follow the patient and only treat if symptoms develop. If sarcoidosis is causing organ damage or patient symptoms, then glucocorticoids, DMARD therapy, and potentially targeted biologic therapy can be used.

## IgG4-related Disease

Immunoglobulin G (IgG) is an abundant antibody that confers long-term immune protection, in contrast to immunoglobulin M (IgM), which is elevated in the acute infection. Four subtypes of IgG exist: IgG1, IgG2, IgG3, and IgG4. *IgG4-related disease* is defined by the presence

| | Sarcoidosis | IgG4-Related Disease | Granulomatosis with Polyangiitis | Rheumatoid Nodule |
|---|---|---|---|---|
| **Pathology** | Noncaseating granuloma | Increased plasma cell + staining for IgG4 | Necrotizing granuloma | Palisading histiocytes and necrotizing granuloma |

FIGURE 15-2. AUTOIMMUNE INFILTRATIVE DISEASES

of abundant tissue plasma cells secreting IgG4. Plasma cells are the mature B cells that produce antibodies. The plasma cells cause tumor-like infiltration and growth into a variety of tissues. Similar to sarcoidosis, any tissue can be affected by IgG4-related disease, but a handful of presentations are more common:

*Autoimmune pancreatitis* can be caused by IgG4-related disease. Autoimmune pancreatitis accounts for fewer than 2% of cases of chronic pancreatitis. IgG4-related autoimmune pancreatitis often presents as a pancreatic mass mistaken for pancreatic cancer. Diagnosis is made on biopsy, which demonstrates an abundance of plasma cells staining for IgG4.

*Retroperitoneal fibrosis* in IgG4-related disease occurs when a buildup of plasma cells and fibrotic connective tissue occurs in the retroperitoneal area, the area in the abdomen behind the intestines and immediately anterior to the posterior abdominal wall. The retroperitoneum contains multiple important structures, such as the aorta, kidneys, and ureters. Retroperitoneal fibrosis can encroach on these structures and cause kidney failure if the ureters are blocked, or ischemia to the lower extremities if the aortic lumen is decreased in size because of impingement by the fibrotic tissue. The discovery may be made during workup of vague abdominal pain with a CT scan of the abdomen, revealing the retroperitoneal infiltrate. In many cases of retroperitoneal fibrosis, the diagnosis of IgG4-related disease is made on biopsy of the fibrotic tissue.

IgG4-related disease may present with a ***retroorbital tumor*** or ***periorbital edema***. The tumor behind the eye may place pressure on the eye and push it anteriorly. Periorbital edema can be mild or severe to the point where the patient cannot open the eye. It is usually unilateral, but may be bilateral.

## Granulomatosis with Polyangiitis

*Granulomatosis with Polyangiitis (GPA)* is discussed in more detail in Chapter 13, Vasculitis. It is important to consider GPA in the differential when a patient has an infiltrative lesion; it could be a necrotizing granuloma from GPA.

## Rheumatoid Nodules

*Rheumatoid nodules* are infiltrative lesions that can present in any tissue in patients with rheumatoid arthritis. It is unclear how often rheumatoid nodules occur in patients with rheumatoid arthritis, because the nodules often do not cause symptoms and are often found during imaging performed for another reason. Rheumatoid nodules can produce problems if the nodules develop in organs or critical areas, such as the brain or spine. On pathology, the nodules classically have histiocytes and necrotizing granulomas.

## Diffuse Lymphadenopathy

Diffuse lymphadenopathy can be seen in infection, malignancy, and autoimmune disease. Infection and malignancy need to be ruled out whenever a patient presents with diffuse lymphadenopathy; this can be done with lymph node biopsy, cultures, and blood tests. Many autoimmune diseases such as *systemic lupus erythematosus* and *sarcoidosis* can cause lymphadenopathy, but this is not the primary presentation. The following are rare autoimmune conditions with a primary presentation of diffuse lymphadenopathy, summarized in **Figure 15-3**.

### Castleman Disease

*Castleman disease* is a diffuse lymphoproliferative disorder (lymph nodes become more pronounced) thought to be an autoimmune or oncologic disease; it is unclear at this time. The underlying pathophysiology is thought to be excess release of interleukin-6, which is a proinflammatory cytokine. Two types of Castleman disease are recognized. They present differently:

1. *Multicentric Castleman* is rare. It presents with diffuse lymphadenopathy and enlarged liver and spleen (*hepatosplenomegaly*). Usually the patients are middle-aged and present with systemic symptoms

| FIGURE 15-3. RARE AUTOIMMUNE CAUSES OF LYMPHADENOPATHY | | | | |
|---|---|---|---|---|
| | **Castleman Disease** | **ALPS** | **DILS** | **Kukuchi Fujimoto** |
| **Area** | Diffuse or localized | Diffuse | Diffuse | Cervical |
| **Population** | Middle age-elderly and HIV patients | Pediatric | HIV patients | Asian |
| **Pathology** | Atrophic follicles and increased vascularity giving a lollipop appearance | Increase in many different types of B cells (polyclonal) with positive special stains | CD8+ T lymphocytes | • Necrotizing • Histiocytic |

(fever, weight loss). The diagnosis is based on biopsy of the affected lymph nodes, revealing increased vascularity referred to as a *lollipop* appearance of blood vessels. A large proportion of patients with multicentric Castleman have HIV/ AIDs. In the HIV patient population, most cases are caused by Human Herpes Virus 8 (HHV8). At this time, multicentric Castleman disease is divided into HHV8 and non-HHV8 associated forms. If the disease is HIV associated, treatment with highly active antiretroviral therapy (HAART) has shown benefit. Other treatments include immunosuppressive medications, including anti-IL-6 therapy.

2. **Unicentric Castleman,** as the name suggests, is lymph node enlargement limited to one area, as opposed to multicentric Castleman, which has diffuse lymphadenopathy. Often, in unicentric Castleman, the patient is unaware of the lymph node enlargement, which may be found on imaging or physical exam. Unicentric Castleman is less likely to have the systemic symptoms (fever, weight loss) that are associated with multicentric Castleman, and it is not associated with HIV/AIDS or Human Herpesvirus 8, but, like multicentric Castleman disease, the biopsy will show increased vascularity and the lollipop appearance.

## Autoimmune Lymphoproliferative Syndrome (ALPS)

*ALPS* is a rare genetic, nonmalignant, diffuse enlargement of lymph nodes in pediatric patients, caused by a mutation in the FAS gene. The FAS gene is involved in programmed cell death, so the mutation likely leads to cells not dying when they are supposed to and then accumulating in the lymph nodes. Patients will usually have accompanying *splenomegaly* and *cytopenias* (low white blood cells, red blood cells, platelets), usually from autoimmune destruction of the cells. Most patients with ALPS require medications that suppress the immune system to control the decreased red blood cells and platelets, as well as the enlarged lymph nodes. Lymph node biopsy shows polyclonal expansion of B cells (diffuse expansion of a variety of different types of B cells, often seen in reaction to infections or autoimmune disease), in contrast to monoclonal B cells (expansion of one type of B cell), which can be seen in malignancy.

## Diffuse Infiltrative Lymphocytosis Syndrome (DILS)

*DILS* is a multisystem syndrome that affects uncontrolled or untreated HIV patients. The presentation is diffuse lymphadenopathy, including enlargement of salivary glands (and subsequent dry mouth), with pathology showing infiltration of CD8 + T cells. Most cases respond to *highly active antiretroviral therapy (HAART)*; the number of cases of DILS has decreased considerably since the availability of HAART. DILS differs from multicentric Castleman, based on presentation: DILS usually involves the salivary glands and pathology that shows a predominance of CD8 cells, in contrast with multicentric Castleman disease, which shows an increased vascularity, i.e. *lollipop* appearance.

## Kukuchi Fujimoto Disease

*Kukuchi Fujimoto disease* is a necrotizing lymphadenitis (necrotizing enlarged lymph nodes on pathology) with a predominant histiocytic infiltrate. The lymph nodes around the neck (cervical lymphadenopathy) are the most common site. Kukuchi Fujimoto disease is much more common in people of Asian descent. Patients often have systemic features such as fever and weight loss. The enlarged lymph nodes can be painful to palpation. This diagnosis is made on lymph node biopsy, which reveals a characteristic pattern of histiocytic infiltration and necrosis. Kukuchi Fujimoto is usually self-limiting but may require immunosuppressant medication.

## Autoimmune Eye Disease

*Autoimmune eye disease* occurs when the immune system attacks a particular part of the eye, causing inflammation. It is important to know the part of the eye that is inflamed because involvement of certain areas gives a clue to the underlying autoimmune cause **(Figs. 15-4, 15-5).** It can be difficult for a non-ophthalmologist to differentiate the different parts of the eye involved in a patient presenting with a red eye or vision changes; these patients should be seen by an ophthalmologist, who can perform a comprehensive eye exam.

- *Keratitis.* Inflammation of the *cornea* (the transparent covering and most anterior part of the eye)
- *Conjunctivitis.* Inflammation of the *conjunctiva* (the highly vascular layer of the inner eyelid and outside of the sclera)
- *Scleritis.* Inflammation of the *sclera* (the white of the eye)
- *Episcleritis.* Inflammation of the *episclera* (a thin connective tissue layer between the conjunctiva and sclera)
- *Uveitis.* Inflammation of the *uvea* (the pigmented layer of the eye, consisting of the iris, ciliary body, and choroid). Uveitis is divided into 3 types based on the location in the eye where the inflammation occurs: anterior, intermediate (inflammation of

the vitreous), or posterior (inflammation of the choroid). If all sections are involved, the term *panuveitis* is used **(Fig. 15-4)**.

## Treatment of Autoimmune Eye Disease

As in most autoimmune conditions, the treatment depends on the severity of disease judged by the ophthalmologist.

Mild disease:

- Glucocorticoid eye drops

Moderate disease:

- Glucocorticoid eye drops
- Oral prednisone

Severe/vision-threatening disease or recurrent disease:

- Glucocorticoid eye drops
- Oral, IV, or periocular injection of glucocorticoid
- One of the following immunosuppressive agents: cyclophosphamide, rituximab, DMARD therapy, or TNF inhibitor

## *Autoimmune Eye and Hearing Loss*

Rarely a patient will have a *combination* of autoimmune eye inflammation and hearing loss that responds to glucocorticoids (*autoimmune hearing loss*). Autoimmune hearing loss is a rare condition where the immune system either attacks the inner ear or causes a growth that obstructs the ear canal and reduces hearing. Autoimmune hearing loss can present acutely with decreased hearing over the course of days or weeks, either unilateral or bilateral. Often, when the inner ear is involved, the patient may experience dizziness, vertigo, and ringing in the ear. There are 3 syndromes you should be aware of when a patient has the combination of autoimmune eye disease and hearing loss:

1. *Cogan syndrome* manifests as corneal inflammation (*keratitis*) along with hearing loss. The patient develops red, painful eyes about the same time as rapidly progressive unilateral or bilateral hearing loss, sometimes with vertigo and balancing problems (vestibular symptoms). Many of these patients can develop large blood vessel vasculitis. Patients suspected of having Cogan syndrome should have imaging of their aorta.

2. *Vogt-Koyanagi-Harada disease (VKH)* manifests as intraocular inflammation (*uveitis*) and hearing loss. Biopsy reveals a granulomatous inflammation. Uniquely, it is caused by an autoimmune response to *melanocytes* (cells that produce melanin, the skin's pigment). Because of the autoimmune reaction to melanocytes, a distinctive physical exam finding is pigment changes especially of the eyelashes, which turn white (*poliosis*). Patients may also have whitening of the skin (*vitiligo*).

3. *Susac disease* classically is a triad of vision loss, autoimmune hearing loss, and cognitive slowing (*encephalopathy*) **(Fig. 15-6)**. It is caused by swelling of the endothelial lining of small blood vessels (*endotheliopathy*) with micro hemorrhages between the damaged, swollen endothelial cells and resultant damage in the affected areas.

   *Hearing loss.* In Susac disease, hearing loss may not be noticed by the patient, but measuring the patient's hearing ability (*audiometry*) will reveal a low frequency hearing deficit.
   *Encephalopathy.* In Susac disease, the patient may notice slowed mentation and increased confusion. In advanced cases, the patient may be unresponsive. Brain MRI will show *snowball* lesions in the corpus callosum, which is an imaging finding highly suggestive of Susac disease.

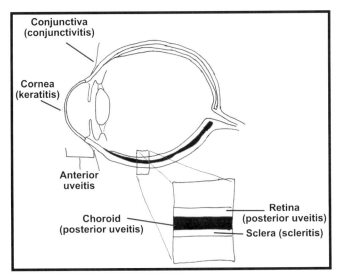

Conjunctiva (conjunctivitis)

Cornea (keratitis)

Anterior uveitis

Choroid (posterior uveitis)

Retina (posterior uveitis)

Sclera (scleritis)

*Figure 15-4.*

| FIGURE 15-5. INFLAMMATION OF THE EYE AND ASSOCIATED AUTOIMMUNE CONDITIONS | | | | | |
|---|---|---|---|---|---|
| Keratitis | Conjunctivitis | Scleritis | Anterior uveitis | Intermediate uveitis | Posterior uveitis |
| RA, GPA, | RA, SpA, SLE | RA, GPA, RP | SpA, Sarcoidosis, JIA | MS, Sarcoidosis, VKH | Behcet's, Sarcoidosis, VKH |

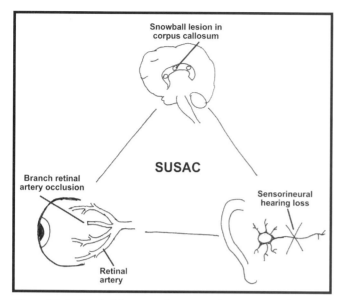

**Figure 15-6.** *Triad of Susac syndrome: autoimmune sensorineuronal hearing loss, vision loss from branch retinal artery occlusion, and mental status changes from lesions in the corpus callosum.*

*Vision loss.* In Susac disease, the patient may notice darkened areas in part of the visual field (*scotomas*). Vascular imaging will show occlusions in the blood vessels supplying the retina, termed *branch retinal artery occlusions (BRAO)*.

## Relapsing Polychondritis

*Relapsing Polychondritis* is an autoimmune condition that targets *type II collagen*, which is found in abundance in *cartilage* as well as the *sclera*. Relapsing polychondritis causes inflammation and destruction of cartilaginous structures, as in the outer ear, nose, upper airway, as well as the sclera of the eye. Relapsing polychondritis is unique among the autoimmune diseases as other autoimmune diseases do not involve the outer ear, so when a patient presents with months of a red/swollen ear (not secondary to trauma), relapsing polychondritis should be high on the differential.

*Ear involvement.* The most common presentation of relapsing polychondritis is inflammation of the outer ear, which is reddened (*erythematous*) and painful to touch. The condition spares the non-cartilaginous part of the ear, the ear lobe. On exam, most of the ear will be swollen and red, but the ear lobe will appear unaffected (**Fig. 15-7**).

*Nasal involvement* includes nasal stuffiness, crusting, and bleeding, which may precede nasal cartilage inflammation. The mid-nose may appear reddened and painful to touch. If left untreated, the destruction of the nasal cartilage will cause a saddle nose deformity

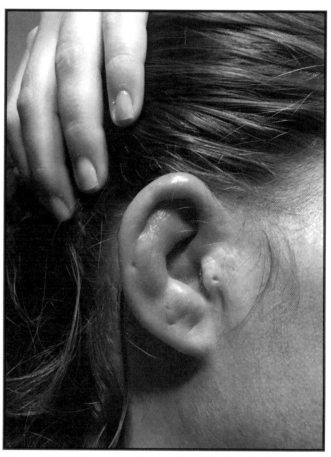

**Figure 15-7.** *Outer ear erythema and swelling in relapsing polychondritis. Notice the ear lobe is spared.*

similar to that seen in the vasculitis *granulomatosis with polyangiitis* (**Fig. 13-6**).

*Upper airway involvement* includes the larynx, trachea and bronchi. The large airways of the lung can become inflamed and actually collapse, severely restricting the airway and leading to hypoxia. Initial symptoms can be changes in voice (hoarseness), wheezing, and possible inspiratory stridor.

*Eye disease* is fairly common in relapsing polychondritis, especially episcleritis and scleritis.

*Joints.* Inflammatory arthritis is a common component of relapsing polychondritis, as cartilage is a major component of the structure of most joints. The inflammatory arthritis seen in relapsing polychondritis is usually nonerosive, as opposed to rheumatoid arthritis, which is erosive.

No blood test exists for diagnosing relapsing polychondritis. Diagnosis needs to be made when a patient presents with the above symptoms. Biopsy of the involved area shows inflammation and destruction of the cartilage.

# Osteoporosis and Osteopenia

*Osteoporosis* is a common condition characterized by disruption of the normal bone architecture, low bone mass, and increased risk of fracture. Osteoporosis is not an autoimmune condition, and it's treated in many different fields of medicine, including internal medicine, family practice, endocrinology, and rheumatology. Rheumatology often treats osteoporosis because one of the largest risk factors for osteoporosis development is a history of glucocorticoid use, which rheumatologic patients often have. Glucocorticoids, most commonly prednisone, can rapidly decrease bone mass and increase the risk of fracture. It is imperative that rheumatologists know about osteoporosis and educate patients about lifestyle and prescription medications that can decrease the risk of fractures while on glucocorticoids.

How is the strength of bone measured? The quantitative measurement of *bone mineral density* (BMD), which is the overall strength of the bone, is by *dual-energy x-ray absorptiometry* (DXA). This imaging study can be done to quantify the strength of a patient's BMD. If you look at the results of a DXA study, you will notice there are lots of different measurements taken, the most important number being the *T-score*.

*T-score* compares your patient's bone mineral density with that of a young and healthy adult. The T-score is the number of standard deviations the density is from that of a healthy young adult of the same sex. The closer the T-score is to zero, the closer the person's bone density is to a healthy young adult's. If it's negative, it means it's less dense, although 0 to -1 is still considered normal. Once the number goes below -1, the person is considered to have low bone density.

## Diagnosis of Osteoporosis and Osteopenia

Osteoporosis is defined by 2 different methods:

1. *Fragility fracture.* A fragility fracture occurs from minimal trauma, such as falling from a standing height. A fracture should not occur if a person falls from just a standing position. Fragility fractures most commonly occur in the spine, wrist, arm, rib, and pelvis. If a patient presents after breaking an arm after falling onto his or her side while walking, then the diagnosis of *clinical osteoporosis* can be made. Clinical osteoporosis means the diagnosis of osteoporosis was made not by imaging, but by clinical history.
2. A DXA scan with a T-score of less than -2.5 is diagnosed as osteoporosis.
   *Osteopenia* is a weakening of the bones, but not quite as weak as osteoporosis. Osteopenia is much more common than osteoporosis and portents a lower risk of fracture compared to osteoporosis, but osteopenia is still not normal.
3. Osteopenia is defined as a T-score between -1 and -2.5.

## Treatment of Osteoporosis and Osteopenia

Anyone with osteoporosis should be treated with medications to reduce the risk of future fractures. It becomes more of a challenge to decide which patients with osteopenia should be treated. One of the tools that physicians use to help decide on treatment for fracture is the *Fracture Risk Assessment Tool (FRAX)*. FRAX looks at multiple variables and then gives a percentage risk of fractures within the next 10 years. The variables that are analyzed include a patient's age, history of previous fracture, history of glucocorticoid therapy, low body weight (one of the few benefits of obesity is a reduced risk of osteoporosis), family history of hip fracture, tobacco use, and excess alcohol intake.

*Bisphosphonates* are usually the first-line therapy for patients at high risk for fractures. In normal bone homeostasis, there is breakdown of old bone and building of new bone. Bisphosphonates decrease the amount of bone that is broken down. They can be given either orally or by IV.

*Denosumab (Prolia)* is an antibody against RANK ligand. RANK ligand is important for the development of osteoclasts, the cells that break down bone. Like bisphosphonates, denosumab decreases the amount of bone breakdown.

*Parathyroid hormone (PTH)* is critical in maintenance of calcium homeostasis within the body. PTH increases the amount of calcium in the blood by removing calcium from the bones. Patients with excess PTH will often have weak bones. It sounds counterintuitive to give a patient with weak bones a protein similar to PTH; however, if PTH is given in intermittent bursts instead of continually, it actually increases the production of cells responsible for the building of bone, called *osteoblasts*. In contrast to the previously mentioned treatments for weak bones, PTH-related treatment builds bone instead of just preventing more bone breakdown.

*Teriparatide (Forteo)* is the PTH-related medication that is currently FDA approved for osteoporosis, and is given as a daily subcutaneous injection. Teriparatide is usually reserved for more severe osteoporosis that is resistant to bisphosphonate or denosumab therapy.

# 16

# *Pediatric Rheumatology*

*Pediatric Rheumatology* is a separate chapter since there are unique rheumatologic conditions seen primarily in the pediatric population. Also, the workup of joint pain in the pediatric population differs slightly since malignancy is higher in the differential for pediatric joint pain than it is for adults. The treatment of pediatric patients with systemic autoimmune conditions also differs slightly since systemic glucocorticoids have more potential side effects in this population.

Most rheumatologic conditions that affect adults also occur in the pediatric population, such as systemic lupus erythematosus and dermatomyositis, with few exceptions (such as Giant Cell Arteritis, which is unique to the elderly population). This chapter focuses on rheumatologic conditions that are unique to the pediatric population or are more common in the pediatric than adult populations.

## Bone/Joint Pain In A Pediatric Patient

### Differential Diagnosis

The differential for joint pain for children and adolescents differs from that of adults **(Fig. 16-1)**. Malignancy as a cause of bone/joint pain is more common in children than adults. Multiple kinds of malignancies should be high in the differential in a pediatric patient presenting with monoarticular joint pain and systemic symptoms, such as weight loss and night sweats.

## Malignancy

Signs and symptoms of underlying malignancy causing joint pain in children include:

- Joint redness (erythema). Redness is rare in inflammatory arthritis in the pediatric population. A red joint in a child should raise suspicion for a septic joint or underlying malignancy.
- Systemic symptoms such as fever, weight loss, or night sweats
- Pain at night as well as during the day
- Enlarged lymph nodes in areas near the affected joint
- Associated bone pain to palpation near the affected joint

*Acute lymphoblastic leukemia* should be considered in any child with painful joints. A blood smear will show elevation in blasts. The patient's complete blood count will often demonstrate anemia and low platelets. The white blood cell count can be low, normal, or high.

*Neuroblastoma* usually presents with bone pain along with systemic symptoms, such as fevers and weight loss. Neuroblastoma tumors usually originate within the abdomen, often presenting with abdominal pain.

*Osteosarcoma* presents as localized bone pain. Occasionally a soft tissue mass can be appreciated around the joint. The metaphysis of long bones is the most common location **(Fig. 16-2)**.

| FIGURE 16-1. DIFFERENTIAL DIAGNOSIS OF BONE/JOINT PAIN IN A PEDIATRIC PATIENT. | | | |
|---|---|---|---|
| | **Symptoms** | **Labs** | **Radiography** |
| **Neoplasia** | Redness, systemic symptoms, pain at night as well as day, lymphadenopathy, focal bone tenderness near the joint | • Leukemia: low hemoglobin, low platelet count. WBC elevated or normal; blasts may be seen on blood smear.<br>• Arthrocentesis: normal WBC to mildly inflammatory | Bone tumors cause bone distortions, ranging from mass-like lesions to poorly defined cystic lesions |
| **Septic Arthritis** | Severe pain, redness, swelling | • Elevated blood WBC, elevated ESR/CRP<br>• Arthrocentesis: WBC 25,000->50,000/mm³; positive fluid cultures in 2/3 cases | Early disease will only show effusion; within days to weeks, x-ray will show loss of joint space and erosions |
| **Inflammatory Arthritis** | • Warmth, limping and/or decreased use of the limb. Redness is rare in Juvenile Idiopathic Arthritis. If more than one joint is involved, the likelihood of JIA is much greater.<br>• Limb length discrepancy: If one limb is longer than the other, this indicates a prolonged disease process. The limb that is longer is often the affected leg, likely because of increased blood flow from inflammation to the joint. | • Elevated blood WBC<br>• Arthrocentesis: WBC 2,000-50,000/mm³ | Erosions can be seen at the articular surface of affected joints if the disease is long-standing. |

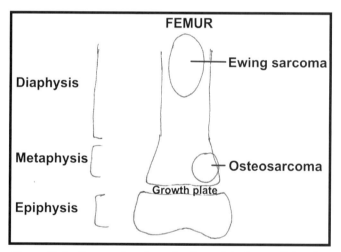

*Figure 16-2.* *Common locations of radiographic abnormalities of two pediatric bone tumors.*

*Ewing sarcoma* is often located in the diaphysis of long bones (femur, humerus) (**Fig. 16-2**), as well as the pelvis. Symptoms present as rapidly worsening localized bone pain.

Radiographs are essential during the workup of joint pain in the pediatric population. A bony neoplasm will exhibit (often not well-defined) distortion of the bone architecture.

X-ray of a *benign* bony lesion may show a variety of patterns, but one of the more consistent benign patterns is a well-defined cystic lesion with a well-defined sclerotic (whitened) border.

X-rays of *malignant* tumors show ill-defined margins with soft tissue calcification around the lesion. If a malignant tumor is suspected, refer to a center with experience in pediatric oncology. MRI will better characterize the lesion and its proximity to nerves and blood vessels (in case of biopsy).

# Workup for Monoarticular Joint Pain in a Pediatric Patient

As in an adult, if a child has a joint effusion, perform an arthrocentesis to better characterize the cause. The synovial fluid white blood count can help differentiate the next steps in workup (**Fig. 16-3**). Crystalline disease (gout, pseudogout) is markedly less common in children than in adults, and it is important to rule out a septic joint, which will usually have a white blood cell count of greater than 50,000/mm³ but occasionally just above 25,000/mm³.

# Autoimmune Arthritic Diseases in Pediatrics

*Juvenile Inflammatory Arthritis (JIA)* is a category of autoinflammatory and autoimmune conditions affecting

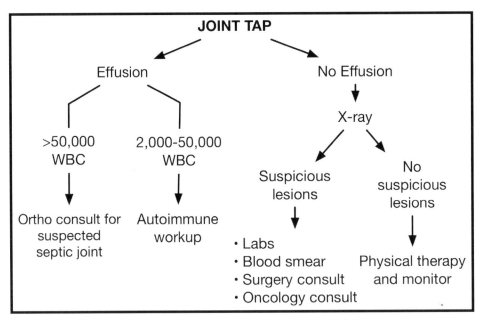

*Figure 16-3. Workup of monoarticular joint pain in the pediatric population.*

the pediatric population. Classifying pediatric patients with JIA can be confusing because the classification system has changed and will likely continue to evolve as the different diseases are better understood. Juvenile idiopathic arthritis is a broad category that encompasses multiple diseases that are very different from one another.

### Systemic Juvenile Idiopathic Arthritis (sJIA)

*Systemic juvenile idiopathic arthritis* is the disease least like the other diseases encompassed in the juvenile idiopathic arthritis nomenclature. It is an autoinflammatory condition, as opposed to an autoimmune disease (the difference is discussed in more detail in Chapter 8, Autoinflammatory Disease). The other juvenile idiopathic arthritides discussed in this chapter are autoimmune diseases. Systemic juvenile idiopathic arthritis is the pediatric form of *Adult Onset Still's disease*. Try to distinguish the remainder of the juvenile idiopathic arthritides from systemic juvenile idiopathic arthritis, and the remainder of the diseases will make more sense.

Systemic juvenile idiopathic arthritis often presents as a constellation of symptoms:

*Fever* is a major component of the patient's symptoms. The classic presentation of systemic juvenile idiopathic arthritis is a daily fever upwards of 102°F, usually in the evening.

*Rash.* A salmon-colored rash often presents along with the fever and often resolves with the spontaneous resolution of the fever.

*Joint pains.* During flares, the patient will often complain of pain and swelling in multiple joints.

*Pericarditis.* Inflammation can also occur within the pericardium, causing chest pain.

Often, once the fever resolves, the more systemic symptoms also resolve. So the patient feels well in between the flares (at least early on in the disease). Autoimmune diseases such as rheumatoid arthritis are usually a daily problem with a steady progression of disease, resulting in a steady debilitation.

#### Diagnosis of Systemic Juvenile Idiopathic Arthritis

No lab test is diagnostic of systemic juvenile idiopathic arthritis, but there are lab abnormalities that can help with the diagnosis. Notably, the ferritin will be very elevated during flares but also between flares. The acute phase reactants (C-reactive protein and Erythrocyte Sedimentation Rate) are also very elevated, especially during acute attacks. In patients with systemic juvenile idiopathic arthritis, *Macrophage Activating Syndrome (MAS)* is an important complication to know about (discussed in Chapter 8, Autoinflammatory Disease).

## Autoimmune Juvenile Idiopathic Arthritis

The remainder of the juvenile idiopathic arthritides are distinguished by how many joints are involved and the presence or absence of antibodies in the blood

(ANA and Rheumatoid Factor). They are considered systemic autoimmune diseases more reminiscent of adult rheumatoid arthritis.

## Polyarticular Juvenile Idiopathic Arthritis

*Polyarticular juvenile idiopathic arthritis (polyarticular JIA)* (previously referred to as *juvenile rheumatoid arthritis*) is classified according to the number of joints involved (5 joints or greater) as well as whether the patient is rheumatoid factor positive or negative. As with adult rheumatoid arthritis, the joints most commonly involved in polyarticular juvenile idiopathic arthritis are the metacarpophalangeal (MCP) and proximal interphalangeal (PIP) joints.

*Rheumatoid factor positive polyarticular disease* usually presents in later adolescence and behaves clinically like adult onset rheumatoid arthritis, even presenting with rheumatoid nodules. Rheumatoid factor positivity and anti-CCP positivity predict a higher risk of joint damage.

*Rheumatoid factor negative polyarticular disease* follows a more benign course compared to rheumatoid factor positive polyarticular disease. RF negative variety is more likely to achieve remission.

## Oligoarticular Juvenile Idiopathic Arthritis

The differential of pediatric oligoarticular (2-4 joints) inflammatory arthritis is broad (**Fig. 16-4**). The labeling of diseases can get a bit confusing, and this is a good example. When we mention oligoarticular JIA, this indicates the patient has oligoarticular inflammatory arthritis that is not caused by SLE or sarcoidosis or an infection. As an example: A child comes in with a swollen right wrist and left ankle and is found to have an asymmetric inflammatory arthritis. This sounds like it could be oligoarticular JIA, but upon further questioning the child has oral ulcers, hair loss, and a malar rash. Then the child would likely have SLE and not oligoarticular JIA. For this section, we're discussing the child who comes in with the oligoarticular inflammatory arthritis and does not have SLE, SPA, sarcoidosis, or an infection.

- Oligoarticular JIA is the most common type of juvenile idiopathic arthritis in developed countries.
- In contrast to polyarticular JIA, oligoarticular JIA is divided into either *ANA positive* or *ANA negative* forms. The difference between ANA negative

| FIGURE 16-4. OLIGOARTICULAR ARTHRITIS. | |
|---|---|
| **Condition** | **Diagnostic Features** |
| Juvenile Idiopathic Arthritis | • ANA+ or ANA −<br>• Uveitis<br>• ENA − |
| Systemic Lupus Erythematosus | • ANA +<br>• ENA+ or ENA-<br>• DS DNA+ or DS DNA−<br>• Multiorgan involvement |
| Spondyloarthritis | • Enthesitis<br>• Psoriasis<br>• Uveitis<br>• Inflammatory back pain<br>• Inflammatory bowel disease |
| Reactive Arthritis | Recent:<br>• Diarrheal illness<br>• URI<br>• Painful urination |
| Lyme Disease | • Tick exposure<br>• + Lyme testing<br>• Rash +/− |
| Sarcoidosis | • African American<br>• Hilar lymphadenopathy on chest x-ray<br>• Tissue biopsy showing noncaseating granuloma |
| Gonococcal arthritis | • Sexual exposure<br>• Fevers<br>• Skin lesions<br>• + Gonococcus in urine, cervical swab, or blood culture |

and ANA positive disease relates to the ocular manifestations discussed later.

- Oligoarticular JIA most commonly involves the large and medium (knee, elbow, ankle) joints.
- The clinical course of oligoarticular JIA from a joint standpoint is more benign than polyarticular JIA, with less erosion and less lasting joint damage. Remission of the joint inflammation often occurs, but the disease can relapse years later, so patients should continue to be monitored.
- The most important morbidity to know about in oligoarticular JIA is inflammation of the eye (*uveitis*), which can lead to permanent visual loss if untreated. The eye inflammation can be asymptomatic, so patients should be evaluated by an ophthalmologist regularly. The largest risk factor for developing uveitis is a positive ANA.

## Enthesitis-related Juvenile Idiopathic Arthritis

*Enthesitis-related juvenile idiopathic arthritis* likely falls more in the category of adult spondyloarthritis (see Chapter 4, Spondyloarthritis). Enthesitis is inflammation in the area where the tendons attach to bone and can occur in a number of sites, but the most common one is the insertion of the Achilles tendon. This differs from inflammatory arthritis, where the inflammation is within the actual joint, more specifically the synovial lining. As in adult spondyloarthritis, enthesitis-related juvenile idiopathic arthritis correlates with *HLA-B27 positivity*, sacroiliac joint tenderness (causing inflammatory back pain), and inflammation of the eye (uveitis).

## Psoriatic arthritis

*Psoriatic arthritis* in children resembles adult psoriatic arthritis. The diagnosis can be made in children with a personal or family history of psoriasis. If a child presents with polyarticular inflammatory arthritis and the child's mother has psoriasis, think psoriatic arthritis.

## Medications in Pediatric Rheumatology

The same medications used in adult medicine are used in the pediatric population, although fewer trials have been done to show the efficacy of these drugs. Systemic glucocorticoids are less used, since their side effects in this population are numerous, including growth retardation, diabetes, bone loss, and elevated blood pressure. If only a few joints are involved, steroid injections can be given to limit the overall exposure to systemic glucocorticoids. Non-Steroidal Anti-Inflammatory Drugs (NSAIDs) can be used in mild disease to limit exposure to glucocorticoids.

Disease-Modifying Anti-Rheumatic Drugs (DMARDs), including methotrexate and a wide range of other rheumatologic medications, can be used safely in the pediatric population.

# Common Non-inflammatory Causes of Pediatric Joint Pain

## Chondromalacia patella

*Chondromalacia patella* is the softening of the cartilage on the underside of the kneecap (patella). The problem is likely caused by improper tracking of the patella during knee flexion. Usually the muscle above the patella (quadriceps) pulls the patella straight upwards during flexion, but in chondromalacia, the patella may track laterally, which allows the patella to grind against the femur. The patient will complain of slowly worsening pain in the knee during activities or prolonged sitting. The pain usually occurs when the knee is flexed.

## Osgood-Schlatter disease

*Osgood-Schlatter disease* refers to inflammation around the tibial tubercle. This condition usually occurs in adolescents participating in sports. It presents with activity as pain over the tibial tubercle, where the patellar tendon inserts (**Fig. 16-5**). Repeated traction on the developing tibial tubercle may cause self-limiting damage until bone maturity occurs.

## Slipped Capital Femoral Epiphysis

*Slipped capital femoral epiphysis* is a common cause of hip pain in a (usually obese) child. The capital epiphysis slips away from the femur along the growth plate, causing hip (usually groin) pain. The x-ray is classically described as the ice cream slipping off a cone (**Fig. 16-6**).

## Legg-Calve-Perthes Disease

*Legg-Calve-Perthes disease* is avascular necrosis of the femoral head in children between the ages of 4-5. The growth of the bone outperforms the supply of blood vessels, and the bone begins to weaken and die (*osteonecrosis*). X-ray shows flattening of the femoral head. Remember it by Legg-CAVE-Perthes, with a "cave in" of the femoral head *(Fig. 16-7).*

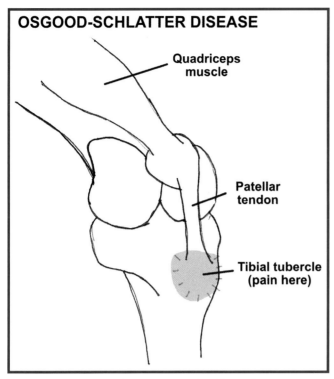

*Figure 16-5. The area of pain in Osgood-Schlatter disease.*

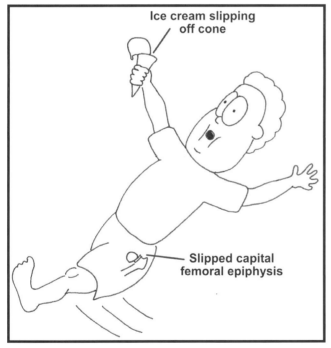

*Figure 16-6. An obese child slipping (slipped capital femoral epiphysis) while holding an ice cream cone (x-ray of the hip appears like an ice cream slipping off its cone).*

## Pediatric Vasculitis

For a more detailed discussion of vasculitis, see Chapter 13, Vasculitis.

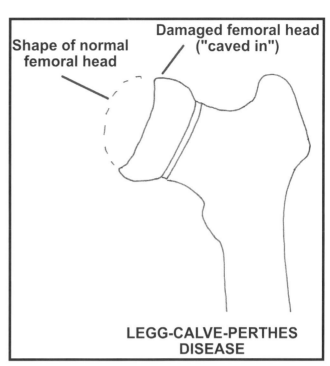

*Figure 16-7. Remember Legg-Calve-Perthes disease as Legg-CAVE-Perthes disease, as the femoral head appears CAVED in.*

### IgA Vasculitis (Henoch-Schönlein Purpura)

*Henoch-Schönlein Purpura* is the most common vasculitis in pediatrics, but it can occur in adults. Think about this disease whenever you see the combination of a young patient with

- palpable purpura (red dots on the skin the examiner can feel, and lesions that don't blanch with pressure)
- abdominal pain
- joint pains

The diagnosis is most often made when biopsying the rash, and immunofluorescence stains show deposition of IgA. The kidneys can be involved in IgA vasculitis; the patient will have blood in the urine and possibly an elevated creatinine. Like ANCA vasculitis, RBC casts may be seen on microscopic exam of the urine. A kidney biopsy reveals inflammation and positive IgA deposition (not pauci-immune like we see in ANCA vasculitis).

IgA vasculitis seems to have a different course depending on whether the patient is young or old, with the pediatric population having more gastrointestinal complications (intussusception and intestinal ischemia), while adults have more joint complaints.

In children, the disease course is often more benign and self-limited, while in adults it can be more persistent and even lead to renal failure.

### Kawasaki Disease

*Kawasaki's vasculitis* nearly always occurs in children, most often between the ages of 6 months and 5 years. Kawasaki is considered a *mucocutaneous lymph node syndrome*, meaning the majority of the symptoms involve the mucocutaneous structures like the mouth, as well as the lymph nodes (lymphadenopathy). Kawasaki's usually presents in children as a recurrent fever of unknown origin along with major oral and ocular symptoms. Symptoms that give a clue are:

- *Red eyes.* Redness is caused by inflammation within the conjunctiva (conjunctivitis) and can be severe.
- *Cracked lips.* The lips may be red, swollen and cracked, leading to severe discomfort of the mouth.
- *Strawberry tongue.* The tongue may turn a deeper red and have small bumps that resemble the skin of a strawberry.
- *Lymphadenopathy. Palpable swelling of the lymph nodes in multiple areas throughout the body.*

The thing to fear about Kawasaki disease is the dreaded complication of *coronary artery aneurysms.* The patient can develop asymptomatic large coronary aneurysms that later thrombose or dissect, leading to death. Any patient suspected of having Kawasaki disease should have an echocardiogram evaluation for coronary aneurysms. The treatment for Kawasaki is aspirin and intravenous immunoglobulin.

# Cases

1. HISTORY: A 4-year-old girl is brought into clinic because of persistent limping in the morning. She doesn't really complain about pain, but her parents noticed the limping and mild swelling of her right knee in the morning, which is no longer swollen by the afternoon. She doesn't have any other complaints. She has no recent outdoor exposure.

   PHYSICAL EXAM: You note mild effusion in the left knee and also a mild effusion in the left wrist, but she has good range of motion of the joints.

   LABS: Arthrocentesis is attempted, but no fluid could be obtained. Erythrocyte sedimentation rate and C-reactive protein are both mildly elevated. ANA is positive, but the Anti-Smith, Anti-SSA/ SSB, Anti-Chromatin, Anti-RNP and Anti-Double-Stranded DNA are negative. Rheumatoid Factor and Anti-CCP are also negative. X-rays of the wrist and knee reveal no abnormalities. The remainder of her labs are normal.

   DIAGNOSIS: She has swelling in 2 joints, the left knee and the left wrist, which puts her in the oligoarticular (2-4) category. Her presentation is consistent with oligoarticular juvenile idiopathic arthritis in the setting of positive ANA and no other symptoms suggesting infection or malignancy (fever, night sweats, weight loss, or fatigue).

   TREATMENT: Have the patient evaluated by an ophthalmologist to evaluate for asymptomatic uveitis. As for the treatment of her joint pains, her symptoms overall are mild and can potentially be treated with nonsteroidal anti-inflammatory drugs (NSAIDs) or as needed intra-articular steroid injections.

2. HISTORY: A 7-year-old boy presents with worsening left thigh pain that he feels is close to his knee. He describes the pain as a "deep ache" that he notices throughout the day and at night. Activity doesn't make much of a difference in the pain level. He hasn't tried Tylenol or NSAIDs for the pain. He's able to use his knee without any difficulty, but standing on the leg causes some pain in the area. In the last few days he's developed a fever at night as well as increased fatigue.

   PHYSICAL EXAM: The left knee and hip have normal range of motion. He has a large area of pain to palpation just proximal to the patella on the left distal femur. No lymphadenopathy is appreciated.

   IMAGING: X-ray of the left femur shows a 3 x 3 cm poorly demarcated destructive lesion of the distal femur. The lesion has a moth-eaten appearance.

   DIAGNOSIS: This presentation is concerning for an underlying malignancy. The patient has difficulty standing on the leg as well as fevers and fatigue. Considering the location and x-ray findings, Ewing Sarcoma is likely; but a biopsy needs to be done to definitively diagnose the condition and initiate appropriate management with orthopedic surgery and pediatric oncology.

# 17

# *Antibodies and Other Lab Tests*

By far one of the most confusing aspects about the field of rheumatology is the vast number of laboratory tests and their sometimes less than specific interpretations. In this section, we'll go through some of the lab tests, including the blood tests evaluating for antibodies associated with autoimmune disease.

## Auto-Antibodies

As you can probably guess, the body doesn't normally produce high amounts of antibodies against its own cells. Everyone, though, produces low levels of antibodies that react with their own tissues; but normally, these antibodies are recognized by the immune system as abnormal and are short-lived. The immune system is always making antibodies to a myriad of different antigens, but only a fraction of these antibodies continue to be produced in high quantity. Any given person might have a low level of antibodies to parts of their own body, like their thyroid or nucleic acid (Anti-Nuclear Antibody). This self-antibody production only becomes a problem when something happens in the regulation of the immune system and the body starts producing large amounts. It is often unclear if these antibodies actually cause the disease or are just evidence of dysregulation of the immune system.

## Anti-Nuclear Antibodies (ANA)

*Anti-nuclear antibodies* are attracted to nuclear material in the cell nucleus. They are invariably present in patients with systemic lupus erythematosus (SLE). Every patient with SLE will have a positive ANA test. Thus, one of the most useful findings to prove a patient does not have SLE is a negative ANA. However, up to 20% of the healthy population has a positive serum ANA but no autoimmune disease; thus, the specificity of ANA is very low.

ANAs can also be positive in many other diseases. If a patient has a history of Hashimoto's thyroiditis, he or she will likely have a mildly elevated ANA. ANA can be positive in rheumatoid arthritis, scleroderma, inflammatory myopathy, and Sjögren's disease. Thus, a high positive ANA may point you in the direction of autoimmune disease, but you still have to figure out what disease the patient really has. ANA can also be positive in patients with certain types of infections. Also, some medications can trigger the body to produce a positive ANA **(Fig. 17-1)**. A patient with a positive ANA from a medication does not necessarily have to stop the medication. The medication only needs to be stopped if the patient is experiencing clinical symptoms or lab abnormalities (cytopenias) of a drug-induced lupus.

You may see the ANA test done in different ways, but the most common way in clinical practice is the *indirect immunofluorescence assay (IFA)*. This technique tells you the titer of the antibody if it is detected. Usually you'll see an ANA positive with a titer of 1:40 all the way to 1:1200. The titer shows how much the patient's serum had to be diluted to no longer be able to detect the antibody on immunofluorescence.

| FIGURE 17-1. CAUSES OF POSITIVE ANTI-NUCLEAR ANTIBODIES. | |
| --- | --- |
| Autoimmune Disease | SLE, scleroderma, rheumatoid arthritis, Hashimoto's, autoimmune hepatitis, inflammatory myopathy |
| Infections | Hepatitis B and C, parvovirus B19 |
| Medications | Blood pressure: hydralazine<br>Anti-arrhythmic: procainamide<br>Anti-tubercular: isoniazid, rifampin<br>Autoimmune: TNF inhibitors<br>Anti-hyperthyroid: propylthiouracil<br>Antibiotic: minocycline |

The higher the patient's titer, the more antibody is present in the serum.

The ANA also has a staining pattern. For instance, the test report will say ANA 1:160 with speckled pattern. The staining pattern isn't as important as it used to be, now that we have other tests for SLE and other autoimmune diseases. The one staining pattern that you might want to remember is nucleolar, as this can indicate underlying scleroderma.

## Anti-Double-Stranded DNA Antibody (DS-DNA) and Anti-Smith Antibody

Besides the ANA test, DS-DNA and anti-Smith are the next antibodies you should know when thinking about SLE. Of all the antibodies that we know are associated with SLE, DS-DNA and anti-Smith are the most specific for SLE. Also, of all the antibodies, DS-DNA is the one that is correlated with kidney involvement in SLE. In addition, the levels of DS-DNA can correlate with disease activity in some patients with SLE (the antibody titer of DS-DNA rises when a patient with SLE is having a flare, and then goes down in remission).

## All the Other Lupus Antibodies

Lots of the confusion about the various antibodies in rheumatology stem from the many different antibodies that are associated with SLE. To confuse things more, some of SLE-associated antibodies (e.g. anti-SSA/SSB) can also be associated with other diseases (Sjögren's). These antibodies have individual sensitivities and specificities for SLE, but they are not dramatically different from one another, so it is reasonable to put them into one group. Think of all of the following antibodies as being associated with SLE and (in combination with ANA positivity) increase the likelihood of SLE:

*SLE antibodies:* Anti-Chromatin, Anti-SSA/SSB (Ro/La), Anti-RNP

## Anti-SSA/SSB (Ro/La) Antibody

To confuse things, multiple antibodies have two different names, including Anti-SSA (Anti-Ro) and Anti-SSB (Anti-La). These antibodies can be positive in primary SLE, but they can also be positive in primary Sjögren's syndrome. If these antibodies are positive, you need to look at the clinical context. If the patient's primary complaints are dry eyes (sicca symptoms) and dry mouth, then primary Sjögren's syndrome is the likely diagnosis. If inflammatory arthritis and a malar rash are the primary complaint, then the patient likely has primary SLE as long as the ANA antibody is also positive. Also, remember that Anti-SSA/SSB are the antibodies you need to know about during pregnancy, because they can be transferred to the fetus and cause heart block. (High-yield Internal Medicine Boards question.)

## Anti-Ribonucleoprotein (RNP) Antibody

Anti-RNP is associated with SLE, but it is also associated with Mixed Connective Tissue Disease (MCTD). MCTD is an overlap disorder, meaning it's a mix of certain types of autoimmune disease, namely SLE (inflammatory arthritis and rash), scleroderma (Raynaud's phenomenon and skin thickening at the tips of the fingers), and polymyositis (proximal muscle weakness). All of the patients require anti-RNP to make the diagnosis of MCTD (see Chapter 5, Systemic Lupus Erythematosus for more details on MCTD).

**Note,** anti-RNP positivity does not mean the patient has MCTD. Anti-RNP can be associated with SLE without an overlap of another autoimmune disease. MCTD is only suspected if a patient has a combination of symptoms (inflammatory arthritis, proximal muscle weakness, Raynaud's) along with the RNP positivity.

## Anti-Histone Antibody

Anti-histone antibody is the antibody you hear about for drug-induced lupus. It is also positive in many instances of non-drug-induced lupus (i.e. regular

| FIGURE 17-2. LUPUS ANTIBODIES. | |
|---|---|
| **Lupus Antibody** | **Significance** |
| ANA | If negative, it's not lupus. |
| Anti-DS-DNA and Anti-Smith | If it's positive, probably lupus. |
| Anti-SSA/SSB, Anti-Chromatin | If one is positive, along with ANA, this increases chances of being lupus. |
| Anti-RNP | If patient has symptoms of lupus, scleroderma, and inflammatory myopathy, consider MCTD; but Anti-RNP can also be found in just SLE. |
| Anti-SSA/SSB | If these are the only positive antibodies, consider primary Sjögren's; but if patient has an SLE picture, it could also be primary SLE. |
| Anti-Histone | If negative, probably not drug-induced lupus. |

SLE), so it is not very specific for drug-induced lupus. The sensitivity for drug-induced SLE is, however, moderately high; so if the test is negative, the patient is less likely to have drug-induced lupus.

In clinical practice, all these antibodies can be very confusing to a non-rheumatologist, but it simplifies things to categorize them based on how we use them clinically (**Fig. 17-2**).

## ANCA Antibodies

ANCA antibodies are tested when there is suspicion for small vessel vasculitis, mainly granulomatosis with polyangiitis (GPA), microscopic polyangiitis (MPA), or eosinophilic granulomatosis with polyangiitis (EGPA). The test is actually two separate tests. The *first* one is subjective; neutrophils undergo immunofluorescence and a lab technician looks under the microscope to see if there is a pattern of antibody staining. We look for one of two patterns: *perinuclear* (meaning around the nucleus), which is P-ANCA; and *cytoplasmic* which is C-ANCA. If one of these tests is positive, then we do the more specific *second* test using ELISA. ELISA looks for what the antibody is actually binding to in the neutrophil, namely proteinase 3 (PR3) or myeloperoxidase (MPO). C-ANCA staining pattern is associated with the ELISA test PR3, and the P-ANCA staining pattern is associated with MPO. (See Chapter 13, Vasculitis for more detail.)

## Scleroderma Antibodies

There are many different antibodies for scleroderma, but you only need to know the three antibodies that are the most common and clinically significant. Know that in patients with scleroderma, the organs associated with the most morbidity and mortality are the kidneys and lungs. Each of the scleroderma antibodies carries a different prognosis for either of those organs, so it is important to remember which antibody is associated

with which organ disease. (See Chapter 12, Scleroderma for more details.)

1. *Anti-Centromere antibody.* This antibody is associated with *limited scleroderma* (skin tightening from the tips of the fingers to the wrists but no skin tightening beyond the wrists). Anti-centromere antibody is associated with pulmonary hypertension. Think limited skin, limited lung (only the pulmonary blood vessels are involved as opposed to the lung tissue). Importantly, these patients often also have *telangiectasias* (*spider vessels* on the face from capillary dilatation), esophageal dysmotility, and calcinosis (calcium deposits under the skin that can make hard, painful nodules).

2. *Anti-SCL70/Topoisomerase antibody* (another antibody with two different names) is associated with *diffuse scleroderma.* The word *diffuse* refers to the skin, which is diffusely involved throughout the entire body. Remember, diffuse skin also has the potential for diffuse lung disease. In patients with diffuse scleroderma, the lung tissue can become fibrotic (*interstitial pulmonary fibrosis*).

3. *RNA Polymerase III antibody.* This antibody is associated with rapidly progressive diffuse skin thickening, and the organ that is most often involved is the kidney. In patients with RNA polymerase III antibody positivity, the most feared complication is scleroderma renal crisis (see Chapter 12, Scleroderma).

## Antisynthetase Antibodies

*Anti-Jo-1* is the most common *anti-synthetase syndrome* antibody. There are many other anti-synthetase antibodies, but Anti-Jo-1 is the one to know for this overlap syndrome (Raynaud's, inflammatory myopathy, fevers, thickened and callused mechanic's hands, interstitial lung disease). All the antibodies in this disease subset are directed against different transfer

RNA synthetases. Transfer RNA synthetases are the enzymes that attach amino acids onto transfer RNA (see Chapter 14, Inflammatory Myopathies).

## Rheumatoid Arthritis Antibodies

There are two antibodies you need to know about in the diagnosis of seropositive rheumatoid arthritis (RA). A patient can have either *rheumatoid factor* positivity or *anti-cyclic citrullinated peptide antibody (CCP)* positivity or both and be considered seropositive for the disease.

1. *Rheumatoid Factor.* This antibody is produced in about 85% of patients with rheumatoid arthritis. Rheumatoid factor (usually an IgM antibody) can bind the Fc portion of other antibodies. The sensitivity of rheumatoid factor for RA is high; but the specificity is lacking, since these antibodies can be positive in acute infections, chronic infections like hepatitis C, cryoglobulinemia, and other autoimmune diseases like SLE. We do not think the RF antibody actually causes destruction in the joint, but is probably just a marker of the disease, not the cause.

2. *Anti-Cyclic Citrullinated Peptide antibody (anti-CCP).* This is the most specific antibody for RA. A patient with a positive anti-CCP probably has RA. Anti-CCP is an antibody against citrullinated proteins. This sounds confusing, because it is. Some proteins in the body have their arginine amino acid converted to citrulline via an enzyme, which is a normal reaction that occurs in everyone. For reasons we don't fully understand, the body can produce antibodies to these citrullinated proteins, and the presence of these antibodies is associated with rheumatoid arthritis. Anti-CCP is associated with a more aggressive disease (more erosions on x-rays), but we do not think the anti-CCP antibody actually causes the joint damage.

## Other Rheumatologic Lab Tests

Rheumatologists love to order and discuss *inflammatory markers.* The two main inflammatory markers are *Erythrocyte Sedimentation Rate (ESR)* and *C-reactive protein.* It is important to note that neither of these tests is diagnostic of anything in particular. Rheumatologists use them to follow patients to see if their particular treatments are helping. For instance, a patient with active rheumatoid arthritis may have an elevated Erythrocyte Sedimentation Rate and C-reactive protein prior to initiating treatment; after treatment is started and labs are rechecked, the inflammatory markers may be normal. If the patient

again starts developing pain and the inflammatory markers are elevated, it likely indicates the disease is not adequately controlled. Conversely, some patients with swollen joints with clearly active disease will have normal inflammatory markers. In this situation, it would not be useful to continue checking these markers on them.

1. *Erythrocyte Sedimentation Rate (ESR)* is a simple test that has been around for decades. A patient's blood is placed into a tall tube that has an anticoagulant in it. The blood is left to sit in the tube for 1 hour. After the hour, the red blood cells will settle at different levels depending on what is occurring with the patient. In a normal patient, the red blood cells will not settle far after 1 hour (a normal ESR). If the patient has an active infection, or active inflammation from an autoimmune disease, the red blood cells may settle further down the tube **(Fig. 17-3).**

Why does this happen? Red blood cells naturally have a slight negative charge around their surface that repels one cell from another. If you place the normal blood of a patient into the tube, the red blood cells will repel one another and stay afloat. The red blood cells settle more in inflammatory states because of elevations in *acute phase proteins* circulating in the body. The body makes acute phase proteins during inflammation from various causes. Fibrinogen is one of the more abundant acute phase proteins and is positively charged, which can interfere with the negatively charged red blood cells. When this happens, the red blood cells will lose their negative charge, aggregate together, and then settle more easily in the tube **(Fig. 17-4).** The patients will then have a higher ESR because the red blood cells will have dropped further down the tube

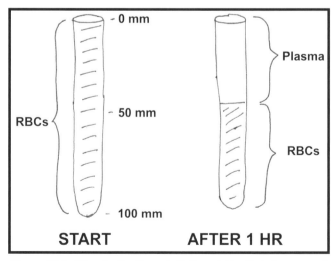

*Figure 17-3. How the Erythrocyte Sedimentation Rate is measured.*

after 1 hour. High amounts of antibodies (usually positively charged) in the blood can also elevate a patient's ESR. Multiple myeloma is an example of a malignancy associated with elevations in the amount of antibodies in the blood with subsequent elevations in the patient's ESR.

The ESR is not specific; things like obesity and a patient's age can give a falsely elevated ESR.

2. *C-reactive protein* is an acute phase protein that is produced by the liver. In active inflammation, whether from malignancy, infection, or autoimmune disease, the amount of C-reactive protein in the patient's blood rises.

C-reactive protein is less likely to be falsely elevated from age or obesity compared to ESR. Of note, C-reactive protein also rises and comes down faster compared to ESR; so when you have an elevated ESR and a normal C-reactive protein, it may be because of the timing the blood was drawn in relation to the inflammatory event.

**Figure 17-5** summarizes the antibodies associated with rheumatologic diseases.

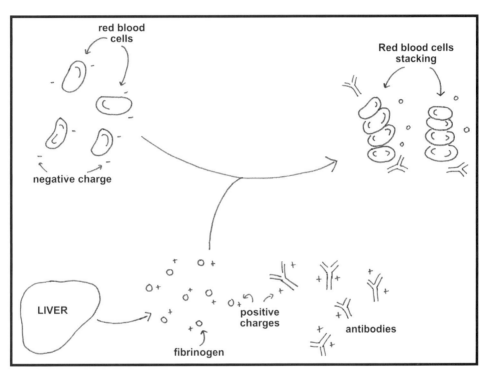

*Figure 17-4. Mechanism of increased Erythrocyte Sedimentation Rate (ESR). Normally, red blood cells repel one another because of negative charges. If something cancels the negative charge, such as positively charged fibrinogen or excess positively charged antibodies, the red blood cells will clump and fall faster, increasing the ESR.*

| FIGURE 17-5. ANTIBODIES ASSOCIATED WITH RHEUMATOLOGIC DISEASES | |
|---|---|
| **Name of Disease** | **Antibody Associated with the Disease** |
| ANCA-associated vasculitis | • C-ANCA associated with granulomatosis with polyangiitis (GPA)<br>• P-ANCA associated with microscopic polyangiitis (MPA)<br>• Eosinophilic granulomatosis with polyangiitis (EGPA) |
| Anti-Phospholipid Antibody syndrome | Beta-2-glycoprotein<br>Anti-cardiolipin<br>Lupus anticoagulant |
| Systemic Lupus Erythematosus | ANA<br>Anti-Smith<br>Anti-DS-DNA<br>Anti-Chromatin<br>Anti-SSA(Ro)/SSB(La)<br>Anti-RNP |
| Sjögren's syndrome | Anti-SSA<br>Anti-SSB |
| Inflammatory myopathy | Anti-SRP: severe necrotizing myopathy<br>Anti-HMG-CoA: severe necrotizing myopathy associated with statin use<br>Anti-JO-1: anti-synthetase syndrome<br>Anti-PL-7: anti-synthetase syndrome<br>Anti-Pl-12: anti-synthetase syndrome<br>Anti-EJ: anti-synthetase syndrome<br>Anti-OJ: anti-synthetase syndrome<br>Anti-KS: anti-synthetase syndrome<br>Anti-Mi-2: classic dermatomyositis, usually mild disease with a good prognosis<br>Anti-MDA-5: amyopathic dermatomyositis (skin changes of dermatomyositis but no muscle weakness) with severe interstitial lung disease<br>Anti-p155/140: dermatomyositis with high risk of underlying malignancy<br>Anti-PMSl: dermatomyositis and polymyositis<br>Anti-SAE: dermatomyositis with mild interstitial lung disease |
| Scleroderma | Anti-Centromere: limited scleroderma and pulmonary hypertension<br>Anti-SCL-70 (Topoisomerase): diffuse scleroderma and interstitial lung disease<br>Anti-RNA-polymerase III: diffuse scleroderma with scleroderma renal crises<br>Anti-PM-SCL: scleroderma and inflammatory myopathy<br>Anti-CENPA-A<br>Anti-CENP-B<br>Anti-RP155 |

# Rheumatology Review Questions

1. **Which of the following presentations suggests NON-inflammatory joint pain?**
   A. 17-year-old with progressively worsening swollen left knee, erythematous and warm to the touch. Cannot bear weight on the knee and has a fever of 101°F.
   B. 55-year-old man with severe pain in the great toe that occurs in the middle of the night, and the patient cannot step on the foot or let a cloth from the bedspread touch the toe.
   C. 30-year-old female with erythematous and swollen MCPs that are stiff in the morning for 3 hours.
   D. 70-year-old man with a dull ache in the distal interphalangeal joints of all digits; pain worsens with activity.

2. **Which of the following locations of joint involvement is consistent with spondyloarthritis?**
   A. The carpometacarpal joint
   B. The temporomandibular joint
   C. The distal interphalangeal joint
   D. The glenohumoral joint

3. **Which of the following characteristics of synovial fluid is concerning for an inflammatory arthritis such as rheumatoid arthritis?**
   A. A white blood cell count of 14,000 cells/mm$^3$
   B. A white blood cell count of 75,000 cells/mm$^3$
   C. A white blood cell count of 500 cells/mm$^3$

4. **Which of the following imaging modalities should be ordered first when evaluating a patient with hand pain in the metacarpophalangeal joints, concerning for rheumatoid arthritis?**
   A. X-ray
   B. Ultrasound
   C. CT scan
   D. MRI

5. **Hydroxychloroquine (plaquenil) is a medication used in a variety of autoimmune conditions. It is not a potent anti-inflammatory medication, but its low toxicity profile makes it an attractive medication to use as monotherapy in mild disease or in combination with other medications in more severe disease. Which of the following is a known toxicity of hydroxychloroquine?**
   A. Liver toxicity
   B. Renal toxicity
   C. Cytopenias
   D. Retinal toxicity

6. **Which of the following clinical presentations is consistent with the diagnosis of calcium pyrophosphate deposition disease?**
   A. 56-year-old man presenting with an acute swollen, painful left knee after undergoing cardiac surgery.
   B. 82-year-old man presenting with intermittent pain in the metacarpophalangeal joints of all

his fingers. Pain is a dull ache with associated swelling, usually lasts 4-5 days, then resolves with taking ibuprofen. Episodes occur every 2-3 months.

   C. 62-year-old woman presenting with fevers, neck stiffness, and elevated white blood cell count.

   D. All of the above

7. **Which of the following laboratory findings is most specific for the diagnosis of rheumatoid arthritis?**
   A. Anti-nuclear antibody (ANA)
   B. Anti-cyclic citrullinated peptide (CCP)
   C. Anti-Double-Stranded DNA
   D. Rheumatoid Factor

8. **Which of the following lab tests is most specific for the diagnosis of Systemic Lupus Erythematosus?**
   A. Anti-Smith
   B. Anti-Histone
   C. Anti-chromatin
   D. Anti-Jo-1

9. **Which of the following are physical exam or imaging findings of osteoarthritis?**
   A. Marginal zone erosions of the metacarpophalangeal joints
   B. Bony enlargement of the distal inter-phalangeal joints
   C. Diffuse swelling of the entire finger (dactylitis)
   D. Swan neck deformities of the fingers
   E. Peri-articular erosion of the metatarsophangeal joint of the 1st toe
   F. Ulnar deviation of the metacarpophalangeal joints

10. **A 25-year-old man presents with a 3-month history of progressive weakness of his arms and legs. He initially noticed difficulty combing his hair in the morning, as he couldn't hold his arms above his head for extended periods because of weakness. The patient also notes difficulty standing from a seated position because of proximal leg muscle weakness. On exam, he has normal strength in his wrists, hands, ankles, and toes. He says he has no pain, just weakness. His serum creatine kinase is found to be greater than 10,000 U/L. Which of the following diagnoses is most likely?**
   A. Polymyalgia Rheumatica (PMR)
   B. Multiple Sclerosis
   C. Guillain-Barré syndrome
   D. Polymyositis

11. **A 75-year-old man presents with a 3-week history of chronic right-sided temporal headache. In the** last few days, he has had difficulty chewing his food because his jaw feels fatigued and painful as he chews. He denies any visual symptoms. On labs, his Erythrocyte Sedimentation Rate is 110 mm/hr (normal less than 20 mm/hr) and C-reactive protein is 5.5 mg/L (normal less than 1 mg/L). What is the next best step?
   A. NSAID treatment for headache and jaw pain
   B. Have the patient scheduled for a temporal artery biopsy and decide on initiating steroids pending the biopsy results.
   C. Order oral prednisone 40 mg daily immediately.
   D. CT scan of the head

12. **A 23-year-old African-American woman presents with a multiple month history of a butterfly rash on her face, painful joint swelling in her metacarpophalangeal joints as well as her wrists and ankles. Labs reveal a hemoglobin of 9.7 g/dl, a white blood cell count of 3.2/µl, and a creatinine elevated at 2.8 mg/dl. Her urinalysis reveals a protein/creatinine ratio of 3.2. Which of the following antibodies is most strongly associated with this presentation?**
   A. Anti-nuclear antibody (ANA)
   B. Anti-Ku
   C. Anti-Jo-1
   D. Anti-double-stranded DNA

13. **Which of the following ocular symptoms is most consistent with the diagnosis of ankylosing spondylitis?**
   A. Conjunctivitis
   B. Anterior uveitis
   C. Branch retinal artery occlusion
   D. Episcleritis

14. **A 23-year-old Caucasian man presents with sudden onset hemoptysis. He noted 4 months of difficult-to-control nasal congestion as well as hearing loss in the left ear, and 3 weeks of migratory joint pain. His chest x-ray shows diffuse opacities and oxygen saturation of 87% on room air. His white blood cell count is elevated; his hemoglobin is low at 8.2 g/dl; and his creatinine is elevated at 3.5 mg/dl with 3+ blood in his urine. Bronchoscopy is performed, and bronchial alveolar lavage shows no evidence of infection. Which of the following labs are most consistent with diagnosis?**
   A. P-ANCA, MPO
   B. Anti-Mi2
   C. C-ANCA, PR3
   D. Anti-CCP

15. A 54-year-old Caucasian male presents with acute onset of right 1st metatarsal phalangeal joint swelling and pain that has progressed rapidly over hours since waking up this morning. The pain is severe, and he can't put weight on the foot. He denies fevers or any other joint involvement. He does note eating a large tray of lobster and shrimp the night before. You suspect gout and perform an arthrocentesis. Which of the following synovial fluid findings are consistent with the diagnosis of gout?
    A. White blood cell count of 600 cells/μL
    B. Negatively birefringent, needle-shaped crystals
    C. Positively birefringent, rhomboid-shaped crystals
    D. Negatively birefringent, rhomboid-shaped crystals
    E. Positively birefringent, needle-shaped crystals

16. A 16-year-old sexually active female presents with a 3-day history of left ankle and right wrist swelling and pain. She has a fever and noticed a painless red bump forming close to her elbow. On physical exam, you note pain radiating down the back of the hand when she extends her wrist against your hand. She also notes recently starting her period. Which of the following diagnostic tests would have the highest diagnostic yield?
    A. Cervical swab
    B. Testing for Lyme antibodies
    C. Serum HLA-B27
    D. Arthrocentesis

17. A 32-year-old woman presents with 3 weeks of progressive joint pain in her metacarpal and proximal phalangeal joints. She notices some warmth and swelling in the joints. Besides her hands, she has no other joints complaints, just mild fatigue. Laboratory evaluation notes mild elevations in inflammatory markers and a slight decrease in hemoglobin. The patient works as a second grade teacher and notes a few of her kids have had to miss class because of illness. Which of the following is the most likely diagnosis?
    A. Rheumatoid arthritis
    B. Lyme disease
    C. Parvovirus-B19
    D. Chikungunya

18. A 62-year-old woman with a history of gout and chronic kidney disease presents with acute left knee swelling and pain. An arthrocentesis reveals a white blood cell count of 17,000 cells/μL and monosodium urate crystals consistent with gout. Her creatinine is at her normal level of 3.7 mg/dl. Which of the following medications can be used to treat her acute attack?
    A. Systemic glucocorticoids or intraarticular steroid injection
    B. NSAIDs
    C. Colchicine
    D. Allopurinol

19. A 74-year-old patient with severe bilateral knee osteoarthritis presents for evaluation. He was diagnosed with osteoarthritis of the knees when he was in his 50's. The patient had previously completed multiple months of physical therapy. He's tried different NSAIDs, which previously gave him some relief, but they're no longer helping his pain. He's had multiple intraarticular injections of steroids, which also previously gave relief but they're no longer beneficial. The pain is the same as it was before, just with more intensity. He's experienced no new trauma, no sensation of instability of the knee. What is the next reasonable step in treatment?
    A. Narcotics for pain control
    B. Try continued physical therapy
    C. Surgical evaluation for knee replacement
    D. MRI of the knees

20. Which of the following imaging findings is consistent with the diagnosis of osteoarthritis?
    A. Narrowed joint space
    B. Osteophyte formation
    C. Subchondral sclerosis
    D. Subchondral cysts
    E. All of the above

21. A 32-year-old woman presents with a 3-year history of pain throughout her body. She noticed the pain started around the time of the death of her father and has slowly become more and more persistent. The pain is a deep ache in both her muscles and joints, worsening with activity. If she overexerts herself, she feels like she won't be able to move for 2-3 days because of the pain. She has severe fatigue as well as concentration difficulties and fluctuations between constipation and diarrhea. She has a long history of depression. What is the most likely underlying diagnosis?
    A. Systemic Lupus Erythematosus
    B. Fibromyalgia
    C. Inflammatory Bowel Disease (IBD) associated with inflammatory arthritis
    D. Lyme disease

22. A 47-year-old woman presents with a 2-year history of worsening dryness in her eyes and mouth. The eye dryness has become severe enough that she was seen by her optometrist and prescribed saline eye drops to place in her eyes at least twice a day. For most of her life, she had excellent dentition, but in the last year she's getting a number of cavities. On exam, you notice decreased salivary pooling under her tongue and mild parotid fullness bilaterally. Which of the following blood tests will most likely be positive in this patient?
    A. Anti-RNP
    B. Anti-CCP
    C. Anti-SSA/SSB
    D. P-ANCA

23. A 42-year-old woman with a history of Sjögren's syndrome presents because of a persistent left-sided facial fullness. She's had a multiple-year history of Sjögren's syndrome with positive Anti-SSA and oral and ocular dryness. She previously developed bilateral facial swelling before, whenever her Sjögren's symptoms were worse, but it's never persisted this long or been unilateral. Which of the following should be your primary concern?
    A. Flare of Sjögren's
    B. Blocked salivary duct from stone formation
    C. Lymphoma
    D. Allergic reaction to food

24. A 47-year-old woman presents with worsening pain at the tips of her fingers, especially when exposed to cold. Over the last few months she's developed thickening of the skin at the tips of her fingers, making them feel "puffy," with difficulty making a fist. When she is exposed to cold temperatures, it not only makes the finger pain worse, but the tips turn bright white, then blue, then red before returning to her normal skin color. She also notes occasional trouble swallowing. On exam, she has thickening of the skin of her fingers from the tips of her fingers to the dorsum of the hands. There is no thickening proximal to the wrists. You cannot pinch the skin on her fingers. Which of the following pulmonary complications is most common with this presentation?
    A. Interstitial Lung Disease (ILD)
    B. Asthma
    C. Bronchitis
    D. Pulmonary hypertension
    E. Chronic Obstructive Pulmonary Disease (COPD)

25. A 23-year-old woman presents to the emergency room with a headache and severe fatigue. She was recently diagnosed with rapidly worsening diffuse scleroderma. Her blood pressure is 210/130 mm/hg, hemoglobin 7.4 g/dl, and creatinine 3.7 mg/dl. One month ago her blood pressure, hemoglobin, and creatinine were normal. Which of the following is the most likely explanation for her current presentation?
    A. Dehydration
    B. Influenza
    C. Scleroderma renal crisis
    D. Hypertensive emergency

26. A 32-year-old woman presents with a 2-month history of fatigue, fevers, and left-sided arm pain. Symptoms initially presented mildly, with increased fatigue and occasional fevers of 101°F. Over the last few weeks the symptoms worsened. She's getting fevers almost daily now, and her left arm began to ache diffusely. The pain is much worse when using her arm and quickly resolves when she rests it. She has no color changes in her fingers. Her labs are noted to have elevated inflammatory markers and an elevated white blood cell count. On exam, she has a weak left-sided radial pulse compared to the right side. The blood pressure in her left arm is 95/45 mm/Hg compared to the right arm of 134/64mm/Hg. What is the next step in the workup?
    A. Blood vessel imaging of the left arm
    B. CT scan of the chest with contrast evaluating for pulmonary embolism
    C. Echocardiogram evaluating for vegetations
    D. Lyme antibody titers

27. A 24-year-old man presents with a multiple-month history of weight loss, fatigue, and fevers. He has severe abdominal pain and new onset of bloody stools. He also notes left leg numbness and tingling and difficulty moving his left foot up and down compared to the right foot. On exam, he appears cachectic and has diffuse tenderness to abdominal palpation. His left foot reveals sensory loss to light touch from mid-shin downward. He cannot dorsiflex his left ankle against resistance. Labs reveal an elevated white blood cell count and very high inflammatory markers. Imaging of his abdomen reveals multiple aneurysm formation of his mesenteric vessels including his renal arteries with evidence of intestinal thrombosis and ischemia. EMG of the left lower extremity reveals evidence of mononeuritis multiplex. He is also found to be hepatitis B positive. What is the most likely diagnosis?
    A. Anti-phospholipid syndrome
    B. Systemic lupus erythematosus
    C. Polyarteritis nodosa
    D. Takayasu arteritis

28. A 32-year-old man presents to the emergency room with the "worst headache" of his life. Symptoms began suddenly while lifting weight at the gym; the headache involves the area all around his head. No visual symptoms. No weakness or numbness of extremities. No other symptoms besides the headache. He notes drinking multiple energy drinks before going to work out. CT scan of his brain shows no evidence of bleeding and no other abnormalities, but vessel imaging of the brain reveals multiple areas of vessel stenosis in both hemispheres. A lumbar puncture is performed, which reveals normal protein, white blood cell count, and glucose. What is the most likely diagnosis?
   A. Migraine
   B. Reversible Cerebral Vasoconstriction Syndrome (RCVS)
   C. Subarachnoid hemorrhage
   D. Central Nervous System Vasculitis

29. A 31-year-old woman presents with a 4-month history of sinus congestion, nasal crusting, and progressive shortness of breath. Chest CT reveals diffuse ground glass opacities, and her serum hemoglobin is low. Bronchoscopy reveals diffuse alveolar hemorrhage. Her creatinine is elevated at 2.5 mg/dl with 3+ blood in the urine. She is also found to be C-ANCA, PR3 positive. What would you expect to find on renal pathology?
   A. IgA nephropathy
   B. Crescentic glomerulonephritis with immunofluorescence staining positive for igG, IgA, IgM, C1q, and C3.
   C. Pauci-immuno crescentic glomerulonephritis
   D. Linear IgG staining on the basement membrane

30. A 52-year-old woman presents with progressive joint pain and shortness of breath. She was diagnosed with asthma 8 months prior, but feels her inhalers are not working as well now. Her joint pain is also worsening. She notes increased pain and swelling in her wrists and elbows, worse in the morning and better as the day progresses. She also notices some numbness in her right foot, but she feels the strength in her foot and ankle is normal. On physical exam, she has some crackles in her lung bases and mild wheezing in multiple areas. Synovitis is appreciated in her wrists bilaterally. There is decreased sensation in the dorsal aspect of her right foot compared to the left foot; her strength with dorsiflexion of the foot against resistance is normal. Laboratory reveals a serum eosinophil percentage of 25%, with elevated white blood cell count and normal kidney function. Her chest x-ray shows a hazy opacity in the left lower lobe. ANCA testing is negative. Which of the following diagnoses is most likely?
   A. Eosinophilic granulomatosis with polyangiitis (EGPA)
   B. Microscopic polyangiitis (MPA)
   C. Rheumatoid arthritis
   D. Bacterial pneumonia

31. A 31-year-old woman presents with progressive painless weakness in her proximal muscles. She notices difficulty combing her hair in the morning because she can't keep her arms above her head without rapidly fatiguing. She also has difficulty standing from a seated position. On exam, you note she has purple discoloration on her eyelids when she closes her eyes. She has an erythematous, blanching rash around her neck. On the dorsal aspect of the joints of her fingers, she has raised erythematous lesions. Creatine kinase is 13,000 U/L. What would you expect to find upon a muscle biopsy of her deltoid?
   A. Lymphocytic infiltrate within the muscle cells (endomysial lymphocytic infiltrate)
   B. Lymphocytic infiltrate around the muscle cells along with atrophy of the muscles cells near the fascicle (perifascicular atrophy)
   C. Normal muscle tissue
   D. Macrophage infiltrate of the muscle with muscle cell necrosis
   E. Rimmed vacuoles with inclusion bodies within the muscle cell

32. A 24-year-old woman is hospitalized because of worsening shortness of breath and fevers. A few months prior to the shortness of breath, she noticed her fingers changing color when exposed to cold temperatures; her fingers will then turn completely white, then dusky blue, then red, becoming mildly painful. She also noticed some puffiness to her fingers as well as cracks and fissures on their sides. On exam, you note sclerodactyly with a small ulcer at the tip of one of her fingers. You also notice some mild weakness in the proximal muscles of her upper and lower extremities. Chest imaging reveals evidence of interstitial lung disease. Her labs show a creatine kinase of 8,000 U/L. Which of the following antibodies is most likely going to be positive?
   A. Rheumatoid Factor
   B. Anti-Jo-1
   C. ANCA
   D. Anti-Smith

33. A 33-year-old woman from Sweden presents with joint pain and swelling in her bilateral ankles and wrists as well as a cough. She also developed a painful rash on her lower extremities. The rash was biopsied, revealing erythema nodosum. Which of the following is the next best step in workup?
A. ANA
B. Chest x-ray
C. Mono test
D. Anti-CCP

34. A 53-year-old man presents with vague abdominal pain and bilateral cheek swelling. He has difficulty explaining where his abdominal pain is, but notes it's more of a "deep pain." He hasn't experienced any facial pain, but has noticed swelling of his cheeks on both sides, with no mouth dryness or difficulty swallowing. Lab evaluation reveals elevated inflammatory markers, as well as a creatinine of 2.2 mg/dl. A CT scan of his abdomen reveals thickening in the retroperitoneal cavity, with encroachment of the ureters bilaterally, consistent with retroperitoneal fibrosis. CT scan of the chest is unremarkable. He is otherwise non-toxic appearing, with no travel outside of the United States. What is the most likely diagnosis?
A. Sarcoidosis
B. Spondyloarthritis
C. IgG4-related disease
D. *Mycobacterium tuberculosis*

35. A 42-year-old Asian-American man presents with anterior cervical lymphadenopathy and high fevers. He has no other complaints. Lymph node biopsy shows necrotizing histiocytosis. What is the diagnosis?
A. Lymphoma
B. Sarcoidosis
C. Kukuchi Fujimoto disease
D. IgG4-related disease

36. A 35-year-old man presents with pain and swelling of the right ear and mild pain in the bridge of his nose. He noticed the red/swollen right ear a few days ago and thought he might have slept on it wrong, but the swelling and pain seem to be worsening. No hearing loss, no discharge from the ear. Left ear has no pain or swelling. On exam, the outer ear is erythematous and swollen, but the ear lobe appears normal. Examination of the ear canal and tympanic membrane is unremarkable. The nasal bridge feels mildly warm and painful to palpation. No pain with palpation of the sinuses, no nasal crusting. Chest imaging is unremarkable. What is the most likely diagnosis?
A. Granulomatosus with polyangiitis
B. Infection
C. Relapsing polychondritis
D. Sarcoidosis

37. A 54-year-old woman with a 20-year history of rheumatoid arthritis presents to your office with questions about her bone health. She feels her rheumatoid arthritis is under control now, but throughout the last 20 years she's been on and off prednisone quite a bit, and she's worried she may have developed osteoporosis. Which of the following tests can be used to give the best prediction of future risk of bone fractures?
A. Dual-energy x-ray absorptiometry (DXA)
B. X-ray of hands and feet
C. Serum calcium
D. Serum vitamin D

38. A 12-year-old girl presents with progressively worsening pain in her left knee and right wrist. Pain and swelling come and go, usually lasting a few days at a time. The pain is usually worse first thing in the morning, but improves with doing activities. She's taking ibuprofen, which seems to help. She has no other symptoms. She's never been sexually active. On exam, you note a swollen, mildly tender left knee and right wrist. Arthrocentesis of the left knee reveals a white blood cell count of 12,000 cells/μL with no crystals; cultures are negative for infection. Chest x-ray is normal; ANA is positive; rheumatoid factor and anti-CCP are negative. Besides treating her joint pain, which of the following is important to continually monitor in this patient?
A. Ophthalmologic exam
B. Chest x-ray
C. Serial arthrocentesis
D. Repeating ANA every 1 year

39. A 3-year-old girl presents with persistent fevers greater than 101°F. On exam, she has a swollen, erythematous tongue, cracked and bleeding lips, and axillary lymphadenopathy. Her labs show elevated white blood cells and elevated inflammatory markers. What is the most likely diagnosis?
A. Kawasaki disease
B. Systemic Lupus Erythematosis (SLE)
C. Kukuchi Fujimotos
D. Castleman disease

40. **A 40-year-old female with no significant past medical history is recently diagnosed with seropositive rheumatoid arthritis. Which of the following medications is a reasonable medication to initiate to decrease her risk of permanent joint damage?**
    A. Adalimumab
    B. Rituximab
    C. Tofacitinib
    D. Methotrexate

41. **A patient with lupus has become pregnant. She is anti-phospholipid antibody negative. Her lupus has been under good control in the last few months. She is only taking hydroxychloroquine therapy. Which of the following medications should be added to her medications while she's pregnant?**
    A. Aspirin
    B. Azathioprine
    C. Mycophenolate mofetil
    D. No additional medications at this time; just continue hydroxychloroquine.

42. **Which of the following medications works primarily by depleting the B cell component of the immune system?**
    A. Abatacept
    B. Rituximab
    C. Tofacitinib
    D. Tocilizumab

43. **Which of the following medications is contraindicated in a patient with a past history of diverticulitis?**
    A. Tocilizumab
    B. Methotrexate
    C. Rituximab
    D. Certilzumab

44. **Which of the following medications can be used to treat an acute attack of gout?**
    A. Allopurinol
    B. Febuxostat
    C. Methotrexate
    D. Colchicine

## Answers To Questions

1. **D.** Remember, inflammatory joint pain refers to joint pain caused by an immune response within the joint, commonly seen in autoimmune diseases, crystalline disease (gout), and infection. Non-Inflammatory joint pain is joint pain that is not secondary to inflammation within the joint. Osteoarthritis is an extremely common cause of non-inflammatory joint pain and affects most people if they live long enough! Osteoarthritis usually presents as a dull ache in the affected joint that worsens when using the joint, as in opening a jar or typing on a keyboard. **A)** This patient has a rapidly progressive monoarticular inflammatory arthritis with swelling and warmth, but also with fever. This joint needs to be tapped to rule out infection. **B)** This patient's presentation is consistent with gout, an extremely painful cause of inflammatory joint pain. **C)** This presentation is consistent with possible rheumatoid arthritis, a symmetric polyarticular inflammatory arthritis.

2. **C.** The distal interphalangeal (DIPs) joints are typically involved in spondyloarthritis, particularly psoriatic arthritis. The DIPs are also involved in osteoarthritis. **A)** The carpal metacarpal joint involvement is typical of osteoarthritis. **B)** The temporal mandibular joint is not typically involved in most autoimmune conditions. **D)** Bilateral shoulder involvement can be seen in rheumatoid arthritis, but is not typical of spondyloarthritis.

3. **A.** A white blood cell count between 2,000 and 50,000 cells/mm$^3$ is consistent with a non-infectious cause of inflammatory arthritis, such as rheumatoid arthritis; systemic lupus erythematosus; spondyloarthritis; and crystalline disease, like gout. **C)** A white blood cell count below 2,000 cells/μL is consistent with a non-inflammatory cause such as osteoarthritis, while a white blood cell count of greater than 50,000 cells/μL **(B)** is concerning for a septic joint, and infection needs to be ruled out.

4. **A.** An x-ray should be the first imaging modality utilized in working up a patient for inflammatory arthritis. X-rays are quick and relatively inexpensive, with minimal radiation exposure to the patient. Importantly, x-rays can also detect other causes of pain, such as a fracture or joint dislocation. Early in the disease, the x-ray may be normal, but it's important to order to rule out other causes of joint pain. Other imaging modalities such as ultrasound and MRI **(B and D)** can actually detect inflammation within the synovial lining (*synovitis*), which an x-ray cannot detect. Most patients with suspected autoimmune inflammatory arthritis presenting with synovitis do not need the advanced imaging of ultrasound or MRI because synovitis can be appreciated on physical exam. MRI and ultrasound should be utilized in cases where the diagnosis is unclear and the physical exam findings of synovitis aren't clear (it may be difficult to tell if a joint is

swollen in an obese patient, for instance). **C)** CT scans are less often ordered in patients with inflammatory arthritis as they do not provide information about tissue swelling.
A. X-ray
B. Ultrasound
C. CT scan
D. MRI

5.  **D.** Retinal toxicity is one of the more concerning side effects of hydroxychloroquine that patients should be aware of. The retinal changes occur over the course of years and are usually preventable and reversible if the patient is evaluated yearly by an ophthalmologist, who can evaluate for the retinal changes seen with hydroxychloroquine toxicity before the patient experiences any vision symptoms. If retinal changes are appreciated by the ophthalmologist, the drug can be stopped, and hopefully the retinal changes will resolve and the patient will never experience vision loss. **(A,B,C)** Liver toxicity, renal toxicity, and cytopenias are generally not seen with hydroxychloroquine, but are potential toxicities of disease-modifying anti-rheumatic drugs (DMARDs) such as methotrexate and sulfasalazine.

6.  **D.** All of the above. Remember, calcium pyrophosphate deposition disease (CPPD) can mimic many different diseases. A patient may present with an acute monoarticular arthritis mimicking gout; hence, the name pseudogout. When this knee is tapped, the synovial fluid will show a white blood cell count usually in the range of 2,000-50,000 cells/µL but will also show positively birefringent, rhomboid-shaped crystals. This contrasts with gout, which demonstrates negatively birefringent needle-shaped crystals. CPPD can also present with a symmetric, polyarticular inflammatory arthritis, mimicking rheumatoid arthritis. One clue distinguishing CPPD from rheumatoid arthritis is the intermediate nature of the pain, whereas in rheumatoid arthritis the joint pain usually is more persistent. **C)** CPPD can involve the neck, causing fevers and a high white blood count, mimicking infectious meningitis. This presentation is called the *crowned dens syndrome* and can be diagnosed on CT scan of the cervical spine, which reveals chondrocalcinosis around the dens of C1. A lumbar puncture will be normal, giving a clue that the neck stiffness and fever is not caused by meningitis.

7.  **B.** Anti-cyclic citrullinated peptide (CCP) is the most specific test for the diagnosis of rheumatoid

arthritis. If you have a patient with joint pain and a positive CCP, then your suspicion should be highly raised for rheumatoid arthritis. Rheumatoid factor is also associated with rheumatoid arthritis, but it can also be positive in a number of other conditions, such as hepatitis C and cryoglobulenemia. Anti-nuclear antibody (ANA) is highly sensitive for systemic lupus erythematosus, to the point that if the test is negative, then the patient almost surely does not have systemic lupus erythematosus. The ANA; however, is very non-specific, meaning many people who have ANA positivity do not have systemic lupus erythematosus. Anti-double-stranded DNA antibody is more specific for systemic lupus erythematosus and is associated with lupus nephritis. If a patient has joint pains and a positive anti-double-stranded DNA, then the suspicion for systemic lupus erythematosus should be much higher.

8.  **A.** Anti-Smith is the most specific test for systemic lupus erythematosus (SLE) listed in the options. Anti-double-stranded DNA is also highly specific for the diagnosis of SLE. Anti-chromatin is associated with SLE, but its specificity isn't as high as Anti-Smith or Anti-double-stranded DNA. Anti-histone is associated with SLE and it's also sensitive for drug-induced SLE. Anti-Jo-1 is an antibody specific for anti-synthetase syndrome, not SLE.

9.  **B.** Bony enlargement of the distal interphalangeal joints is consistent with a *Heberden's node*, a physical exam finding for osteoarthritis. If the bony enlargement is appreciated on the proximal interphalangeal joint, this is referred to as a *Bouchard's node*, also found in osteoarthritis. Bony enlargement of the metacarpal phalangeal joints is much less commonly seen in osteoarthritis. **A)** Marginal zone erosions of the metacarpophalangeal joints are classically seen in rheumatoid arthritis. **D)** and **F)** The physical exam findings of swan neck deformities as well as ulnar deviation of the metacarpal phalangeal joints are consistent with the diagnosis of rheumatoid arthritis. **C)** Diffuse swelling of a finger or a toe (dactylitis) is typically seen in spondyloarthritis, such as ankylosing spondylitis or psoriatic arthritis. **E)** Peri-articular erosions (meaning erosions near the joint, but not within the joint) are typically seen in gout.

10. **D.** This patient is most likely presenting with polymyositis, an inflammatory myopathy. He is weak because of autoimmune inflammation of the proximal muscles with destruction of the muscles.

The condition is usually painless and associated with very high elevations in serum creatine kinase. A definitive diagnosis can be made with a muscle biopsy of a proximal muscle. If this is polymyositis, the muscle biopsy will demonstrate endomysial lymphocytic inflammation. This patient's presentation can also be seen in other inflammatory myopathies, such as necrotizing myopathy and dermatomyositis, although dermatomyositis usually presents with skin findings as well. The types of inflammatory myopathy can be distinguished by the muscle biopsy. **A)** Polymyalgia rheumatica is the inflammatory condition that causes bilateral shoulder and upper thigh pain in people over age 50, with most people developing the condition in their 70's. PMR symptoms are predominated by pain and stiffness in the shoulders and thighs, not weakness. PMR also almost always has elevations in serum inflammatory markers, but not elevations in serum creatine kinase. PMR presents with proximal muscle pain, whereas polymyositis presents with proximal muscle weakness without pain. Patients with multiple sclerosis **(B)** can present with weakness but usually also have sensory loss, including vision changes (optic neuritis). We wouldn't expect the CK to be this elevated in multiple sclerosis. **C)** Guillain-Barré syndrome is a symmetric ascending sensory loss usually associated with a recent infection or vaccination. Again, we wouldn't expect such an elevated CK in Guillain-Barré syndrome.

11. **C.** This patient has symptoms highly concerning for Giant Cell Arteritis (GCA). If left untreated, he is at risk for developing permanent vision loss. Giant Cell Arteritis is a large-vessel vasculitis that exclusively affects people above the age of 50, the majority with elevated inflammatory markers, presenting with either new headaches or pain in the jaw on eating (jaw claudication). If left untreated, the concerning risk is development of permanent vision loss in one or both eyes. When GCA is suspected, high-dose prednisone should be initiated immediately to dramatically reduce the risk of vision loss. **B)** The diagnosis can be proven with a temporal artery biopsy, which will remain positive for multiple weeks even in patients already on prednisone. **A and D)** NSAIDs or a CT scan of the head may eventually be ordered in a patient with new onset headache, but at this point GCA needs to be evaluated and ruled out as much as possible before proceeding with an alternative headache workup.

12. **D.** Anti-Double-Stranded DNA is the antibody most specific for systemic lupus erythematosus (SLE). It is also the most associated with lupus nephritis, which this patient most likely has, considering her high urine protein levels. **A)** Anti-nuclear antibody (ANA) is highly sensitive for SLE but it's not specific. Anti-Double-Stranded DNA is more associated with lupus nephritis than the ANA. **B)** Anti-Ku is associated with inflammatory myopathy, and **(C)** anti-Jo-1 is associated with anti-synthetase antibody.

13. **B.** Ankylosing spondylitis is the spondyloarthritis most commonly associated with anterior uveitis. Remember, inflammation within the eye can occur in a number of different areas, and the different areas can give clues to the underlying diagnosis. **A)** Conjunctivitis is associated with reactive arthritis, but also a majority of viral illnesses. **C)** Branch retinal artery occlusion is associated with Susac Syndrome, and **(D)** episcleritis can be seen in patients with rheumatoid arthritis and ANCA-associated vasculitis.

14. **C.** This presentation is most consistent with granulomatosis with polyangiitis (GPA), which is associated most strongly with C-ANCA, PR3 positivity. The pulmonary opacities are most likely diffuse alveolar hemorrhage, which explains the low hemoglobin; and the acute kidney injury is most likely rapidly progressive glomerulonephritis, which is hinted at by the blood in the urine. A kidney biopsy can confirm the diagnosis if it shows a pauci-immune glomerulonephritis. Another ANCA vasculitis, microscopic polyangiitis, can also cause lung and kidney involvement, but lacks sinus involvement and is typically associated with P-ANCA, MPO positivity. Anti-Mi2 is associated with inflammatory myopathy, and Anti-CCP is the most specific blood test for rheumatoid arthritis.

15. **B.** Negatively birefringent, needle-shaped crystals are consistent with uric acid crystals and gout. We would expect a white blood cell count greater than 2,000 cells/mm$^3$ because gout causes an inflammatory joint pain. A white blood cell count less than 2,000 cells/mm$^3$ is consistent with a non-inflammatory joint pain such as osteoarthritis. **C)** Positively birefringent, rhomboid-shaped crystals are consistent with calcium pyrophosphate crystals and pseudogout. The other two options are not associated with a clinical entity.

16. **A.** Cervical swab has the highest yield for diagnosing *Neisseria gonorrhoeae*, the most likely diagnosis in this young, sexually active patient presenting with an asymmetric oligoarticular inflammatory

arthritis, with a cutaneous pustule on her skin and tenosynovitis on exam (pain radiating down the hand with extension of the wrist against pressure). Another clue to the diagnosis is that the symptoms occur during her period, a common time for *N. gonorrhoeae* to disseminate. **D)** Arthrocentesis is a reasonable answer, and it's always good to take fluid out of joint to rule out septic joint, but the question specifically asks which of the listed diagnostic tests will have the highest yield, and a cervical swab has a much higher yield for the diagnosis of disseminated gonococcus than arthrocentesis. **B)** Testing for Lyme is less likely to be useful. Although she does have an asymmetric oligoarticular arthritis, she has had no clear exposure to ticks. Her history is more consistent with disseminated gonorrhoea. **C)** HLA-B27 is associated with spondyloarthritis, which can present with an asymmetric oligoarticular arthritis, but with the acuity of her presentation and her fevers, infection needs to first be ruled out. Also, HLA-B27 has low specificity, so it's not a good diagnostic test.

17. **C.** Parvovirus B19 is a viral mimicker of rheumatoid arthritis. Parvovirus B19 usually presents with symmetric polyarticular inflammatory arthritis in the metacarpal and proximal interphalangeal joints. Being a teacher increases her risk of exposure to children who may have Parvovirus B19, which presents as slapped cheeks disease. Parvovirus can also present in adults with mild cytopenia, which she also has. **A)** Rheumatoid arthritis is a possible diagnosis, but the diagnosis is not usually made when symptoms are present for less than 6 weeks (unless positive RF or CCP), because viral illnesses can mimic rheumatoid arthritis and lead to unnecessary prolonged therapy if treatment for rheumatoid arthritis is initiated. **B)** Lyme disease usually presents with a monoarticular or oligoarticular asymmetric inflammatory arthritis. **D)** Chikunguyna, a viral cause of joint pain, mimics rheumatoid arthritis, as does Parvovirus-B19, but the exposure would be recent—a Caribbean vacation or trip to India, where the disease is more prevalent.

18. **A.** Chronic kidney disease limits the options of treating acute gout. Systemic glucocorticoids such as prednisone can rapidly reduce the swelling and pain associated with acute attacks and can be given in chronic kidney disease. Intraarticular steroid injection can also be given in acute attacks, especially when only a few joints are involved, which makes the injections easier to perform. If multiple joints are involved, it's often easier to give prednisone

systemically instead of injecting multiple joints. **B and C)** NSAIDs and colchicine are excellent options for acute attacks of gout, but cannot be given in chronic kidney disease. **D)** Allopurinol is a urate-lowering medication, given to prevent future attacks. Allopurinol will not help with the immediate pain and swelling of an acute attack.

19. **C.** In a patient with progressive osteoarthritis that has failed conservative management (NSAIDs, physical therapy, bracing, intraarticular injections), surgical evaluation is reasonable, which can be a more permanent therapeutic option. Continued physical therapy and injections are likely to be minimally beneficial in this patient, who has progressive disease over the course of 20 years. Additional imaging is unlikely going to change management; his pain is the same as before, just more intense, without any new joint trauma, which would raise suspicion for ligamentous injury.

20. **E.** All of the above imaging findings are consistent with osteoarthritis. Osteoarthritis usually presents with multiple imaging findings, including asymmetric joint space narrowing due to loss of cartilage between the joints. Bony outgrowths (osteophytes) are usually seen, are often palpable on exam and appear as bony enlargement of the joint. Subchondral sclerosis appears as an increased whitening along the edges of the joint. Subchondral cysts are small, circular-appearing lucencies within the joint.

21. **B.** This patient's presentation is most consistent with fibromyalgia. Fibromyalgia often presents with many symptoms, but the most predominant one is usually diffuse pain or severe fatigue. The pain is usually in muscles and joints and is usually worse as the day progresses. Even the gentle touching of skin may elicit a major pain response from the patient. Also consistent with the diagnosis is the report that symptoms began after a major life event, the death of the patient's father. **A)** Systemic lupus erythematosus may also present with multiple symptoms, but the joint pain is usually a classic inflammatory arthritis history, with joint swelling and pain, worse in the morning and better with activity. SLE usually does not cause specific muscle aches. **C)** Inflammatory bowel disease associated arthritis isn't likely in this patient; she fluctuates between constipation and diarrhea, which is more consistent with irritable bowel syndrome. If she has inflammatory bowel disease, we would expect more persistent diarrhea and possibly blood in the stools.

**D)** Lyme disease presents with a rash after exposure to ticks, and then develops more commonly into a monoarticular inflammatory arthritis, not full body aches.

22. **C.** This patient's presentation is most consistent with primary Sjögren's syndrome. Sjögren's is an autoimmune disease that targets the tear ducts and salivary glands, causing severe eye and mouth dryness. The most commonly associated antibodies are anti-SSA and anti-SSB. **A)** Anti-RNP is associated with systemic lupus erythematosus and, in more rare cases, mixed connective tissue disease. We would expect the patient to have more symptoms if she had either of these conditions. **B)** Anti-CCP is associated with rheumatoid arthritis and **D)** ANCA antibody is associated with small-vessel vasculitis.

23. **C.** Lymphoma should be high on your differential with an unexplained mass in a patient with Sjögren's syndrome. Patients with autoimmune disease have a slightly higher risk of malignancy, particularly lymphoma, compared to the general population, but Sjögren's has the highest association with lymphoma. Patients with Sjögren's often develop fluctuating bilateral parotid enlargement that will feel like facial fullness to the patient, but if the fullness persists and especially if it is unilateral, an Ear Nose and Throat evaluation should be pursued for biopsy. **A), B), D)** All of these options are possible, but lymphoma needs to be ruled out in a patient with persistent unilateral facial swelling in Sjögren's.

24. **D.** This patient's presentation is most consistent with the diagnosis of limited scleroderma. Scleroderma causes skin thickening that may be limited or diffuse, depending on the extent of skin involvement. Skin thickening can be appreciated on exam by pinching the skin on the fingers; if the skin does not tent up between your fingers, this is consistent with thickening and is called sclerodactyly. Patients with limited scleroderma often have other complications such as GI dysmotility, telangiectasias, and pulmonary hypertension. Remember, limited skin, limited pulmonary involvement. In contrast, diffuse scleroderma is associated with diffuse pulmonary disease, interstitial lung disease (ILD). The remainder of the pulmonary options are not typically associated with autoimmune conditions, other than asthma, which is associated with eosinophilic granulomatosis with polyangiitis (EGPA).

25. **C.** This patient's presentation is most concerning for scleroderma renal crisis. Scleroderma renal

crisis occurs more often in patients with diffuse skin disease and also early on in the course of disease, usually within the first few years of skin thickening. Scleroderma renal crisis presents with elevated blood pressure, acute kidney injury, and usually anemia from red blood cell destruction. The treatment for this condition is rapid initiation of ACE inhibitors, such as captopril. Scleroderma renal crisis is the only time that ACE inhibitors are indicated in the presence of acute kidney injury. **A)** Dehydration is unlikely; we would expect low blood pressure in the setting of severe dehydration, as well as a mild increase in hemoglobin because of hemoconcentration. **B)** Influenza would produce fevers and diffuse body aches, which is not her presentation. **D)** Hypertensive emergency can produce acute kidney injury, but we wouldn't expect the low hemoglobin. Also, considering her history of recent scleroderma, scleroderma renal crisis is more likely.

26. **A.** This patient's presentation is most consistent with Takayasu's arteritis. The next best step would be imaging her blood vessels, particularly the left subclavian artery. Blood vessels imaging can be done by MRA, CTA, or arteriography. In Takayasu's arteritis, we will expect some vessel narrowing that limits blood flow and causes symptoms of claudication in her left arm when she uses the arm. An arterial blood clot in the subclavian artery could cause symptoms of claudication, but we wouldn't expect the fevers, fatigue, and progressive nature of her symptoms; a blood clot usually presents more acutely. Lyme disease does not present with extremity claudication, so this wouldn't be an appropriate test to order.

27. **C.** This patient's presentation is concerning for polyarteritis nodosa (PAN). PAN is a very rare medium-vessel vasculitis that has a propensity to involve the mesenteric blood and renal arteries, causing inflammation and thrombosis in these vessels, leading to infarcts in the intestines and kidneys. PAN also involves the blood vessels of the extremities, particularly those of the peripheral nervous system, which causes sensory and motor loss, a mononeuritis multiplex on EMG. PAN is highly associated with hepatitis B infection. There is no blood test to diagnose PAN. **A)** Anti-phospholipid syndrome can present with diffuse thrombosis, which can appear like PAN, but we wouldn't expect the multiple-month history of fatigue and weight loss. Also, anti-phospholipid antibody syndrome isn't associated with hepatitis B.

**D)** Takaysu's arteritis is a vasculitis of large blood vessels, most often the aorta, carotid, and subclavian arteries in young women. Active Takayasu's arteritis can also produce the fevers, fatigue, and weight loss, but we would expect different vessel distribution. **B)** Systemic lupus erythematosus usually presents with an inflammatory arthritis, rash as well as kidney involvement, usually presenting with proteinuria. Systemic lupus erythematosus would be less likely to present with mononeuritis multiplex.

28. **B.** Reversible cerebral vasoconstriction syndrome (RCVS) is the most likely diagnosis in this patient. RCVS is an acute constriction of blood vessels within the brain that causes sudden onset, severe headaches. The episodes are usually preceded by strenuous activity, or stimulants such as high amounts of caffeine that are seen in energy drinks. The vessel imaging of RCVS is identical to that of central nervous system vasculitis; both show areas of narrowing within the blood vessels. Importantly, **(D)** central nervous system vasculitis will have elevations in cerebral spinal fluid protein or white blood cell count or both. Central nervous system vasculitis also does not usually present as acutely as this patient did. **A)** A migraine may present with sudden severe headache, but we wouldn't expect the vascular imaging abnormalities. **C)** Subarachnoid hemorrhage can also present with sudden onset severe headache, but bleeding would be found on the initial CT of the head.

29. **C.** This patient's presentation is consistent with granulomatosis with polyangiitis. She has sinus, lung, and renal involvement. The pathology most commonly associated with GPA is pauci-immune glomerulonephritis. **A)** IgA deposition is consistent with IgA vasculitis, which is rare in adults, and would not be expected to involve the sinuses and lungs. IgA vasculitis usually involves the skin and kidneys in adults. **B)** Lupus nephritis pathology would reveal crescentic glomerulonephritis with positive IgG, IgA, IgM, C1q, and C3. Systemic lupus erythematosus is less likely to cause diffuse alveolar hemorrhage than GPA; also we wouldn't expect a positive C-ANCA/PR3 in a patient with SLE. **D)** IgG deposition along the basement membrane on kidney pathology is consistent with Goodpasture disease, which is an antibody directed against the basement membrane in the kidney and lungs. We wouldn't expect the patient to have sinus involvement with this disease.

30. **A.** Remember, whenever you hear of an adult who develops asthma and then develops multiple other symptoms, always think of the possibility of eosinophlic granulomatosis with polyangiitis (EGPA, formerly called Churg-Strauss Syndrome). EGPA is an ANCA-associated vasculitis, usually P-ANCA and MPO positive; but EGPA, compared to other ANCA vasculitides, is more likely to not have a positive ANCA test, which makes it confusing and more difficult to diagnose. In other words, having a positive P-ANCA/MPO raises suspicion for EGPA, but a negative test does not rule it out. EGPA can involve multiple systems, namely the sinuses, lungs (pulmonary infiltrates and asthma), nervous system (sensory and motor loss of extremities, usually the foot), and joints; but one of its most prominent features is the high number of peripheral eosinophils, which distinguishes it from other systemic vasculitides. This patient's sensory loss in the right foot is concerning for early nervous system involvement, and rapid treatment will reduce her risk of progression to motor loss in the foot. **B)** Microscopic polyangiitis can involve the lungs, but doesn't present with asthma; the classic lung finding in microscopic polyangiitis is diffuse alveolar hemorrhage. Microscopic polyangiitis is also less likely to involve the nervous system and isn't associated with peripheral eosinophilia. **D)** Bacterial pneumonia wouldn't be expected to cause the joint pain unless there is a concomitant reactive arthritis, but also wouldn't be expected to have this degree of eosinophilia unless the infection is parasitic. **C)** Rheumatoid arthritis could explain the symmetric inflammatory joint pain and occasional lung involvement, but wouldn't explain the peripheral eosinophilia or adult onset asthma.

31. **B.** This patient's presentation is consistent with dermatomyositis. She has multiple rashes consistent with the diagnosis: heliotrope rash, shawl sign, and Gottron's papules. She has proximal muscle weakness and elevated creatine kinase. A biopsy in dermatomyositis will demonstrate lymphocytic infiltrate with perifascicular atrophy. **A)** This biopsy would indicate polymyositis, which has lymphocytic endomysial infiltrate. **C)** We would not expect a normal muscle biopsy in a patient with such weakness and elevated creatine kinase. **D)** Macrophage infiltrate instead of lymphocytic infiltrate with muscle cell necrosis is consistent with a necrotizing myopathy. **E)** The biopsy findings of rimmed vacuoles and inclusion bodies is consistent with inclusion body myositis, which presents in much older patients and has both proximal and distal weakness.

32. **B.** This patient appears to present with an overlap syndrome, with lung involvement (ILD), finger involvement (scleroderma and mechanic's hands), inflammatory myopathy and fevers; this is concerning for anti-synthetase syndrome. Anti-Jo-1 is the most common antibody seen in anti-synthetase syndrome. **A)** Rheumatoid factor is associated with rheumatoid arthritis, and we would not expect sclerodactyly to be present in a patient with rheumatoid arthritis. **D)** Anti-Smith is specific antibody for systemic lupus erythematosus (SLE), but in SLE we wouldn't expect to have the muscle involvement and sclerodactyly. **C)** ANCA-associated vasculitis can involve the lung, but less commonly with sclerodactyly.

33. **B.** This patient's presentation is consistent with *Löfgren syndrome,* a presentation of sarcoidosis consisting of joint pains (particularly ankle pain), erythema nodosum, and hilar lymphadenopathy on chest x-ray. If the patient has hilar lymphadenopathy, the diagnosis of sarcoidosis could be made without an additional biopsy. Löfgren syndrome, for reasons not understood, is more common in Scandinavian countries as well as Spain. **D)** Anti-CCP is the most specific antibody for rheumatoid arthritis; she does have joint pains, but it wouldn't explain the erythema nodosum and the cough. **A)** ANA is a sensitive test for systemic lupus erythematosus, but a positive ANA would not make a diagnosis of SLE. Her presentation could be consistent with early SLE, but other conditions like sarcoidosis need to be ruled out, considering that erythema nodosum is more associated with sarcoidosis than it is with SLE. **C)** Mono test would be inappropriate at this time; erythema nodosum can present post infectious but, considering her joint pain and cough, sarcoidosis would be more likely.

34. **C.** This presentation is most consistent with IgG4-related disease, one of the causes of infiltrative lesions in rheumatology. Classically, it can cause retroperitoneal fibrosis, pancreatic masses, and bilateral parotid swelling, but can involve any organ system. Sarcoidosis and *Mycobacterium tuberculosis* can both cause infiltrative diseases but the normal CT scan of the chest makes both of these diseases less likely. **A)** Sarcoidosis almost always involves the lungs, classically with hilar lymphadenopathy. **D)** Mycobacterium tuberculosis also usually involves the lungs, but it can infect outside the lungs as well. The patient doesn't have fevers and has no history of travel abroad, making *M. tuberculosis* less likely.

**B)** Spondyloarthritis is not associated with parotid swelling or retroperitoneal fibrosis.

35. **C.** Kukuchi Fujimoto is characterized by cervical lymphadenopathy, fevers, and a biopsy showing necrotizing histiocytosis. This disease is often self-resolving, but if symptoms persist, glucocorticoids can be administered. The biopsy findings are not consistent with **(A)** lymphoma. **B)** Sarcoidosis would present histologically as non-caseating granulomas, and **(D)** IgG4-related disease would be characterized by an increased number of plasma cells staining positive for IgG4.

36. **C.** Relapsing polychondritis is the most likely diagnosis. Relapsing polychondritis is characterized by cartilage inflammation, most commonly in the outer ear and bridge of the nose. A typical presentation is erythema and swelling of the outer ear, sparing the ear lobe as in this patient. He also has warmth to the bridge of the nose, which likely indicates inflammation of the nasal cartilage. Without prompt treatment with glucocorticoids, he risks developing a saddle nose deformity. Patients with relapsing polychondritis can also have upper airway involvement with subglottic stenosis. This can be assessed with visualization of the upper airway by Ear, Nose, and Throat physicians or pulmonologists. **A)** Granulomatosis with polyangiitis can have nasal involvement like this patient's, but it would be unusual to develop the warmth and swelling of the outer ear in GPA, which is much more consistent with relapsing polychondritis. **D)** Sarcoidosis can involve a number of different organs, but the normal chest imaging makes this unlikely. **B)** Infection would be unlikely to involve one ear as well as the nose.

37. **A.** The best study to diagnose osteoporosis is Dual-energy X-ray Absorptiometry (DXA), which can be done on multiple areas of the body; and a T-score will be given as either normal bone, osteopenia, or osteoporosis. **B)** X-rays may show decreased density, which raises suspicion for osteopenia, but osteoporosis cannot be diagnosed by x-ray. **C)** Serum calcium is not helpful in diagnosing osteoporosis. **D)** Vitamin D levels should be evaluated in the workup for osteoporosis, since low levels increase the risk for future fractures and should be treated, but vitamin D levels do not help with diagnosing osteoporosis.

38. **A.** This pediatric patient has ANA-positive oligoarticular juvenile inflammatory arthritis.

She has 2 joints involved. The synovial fluid is inflammatory (white blood cell count between 2,000-50,000 cells/µL), non-crystalline, and non-infectious. Chest x-ray is unremarkable, making sarcoidosis less likely. She is ANA positive, which increases her risk of developing inflammation in the eye, which can be asymptomatic; but she should nonetheless be evaluated by an ophthalmologist. Repeating chest-ray would not be beneficial. Repeating ANAs every year would not be useful.

39. **A.** This young patient's presentation is most concerning for Kawasaki disease, a pediatric vasculitis. Suspect Kawasaki's disease in young patients with lymphadenopathy and persistent fever of unclear etiology. A swollen and red tongue along with cracked lips can help narrow the diagnosis. Treat with aspirin and intravenous immunoglobulin. The most feared complication is rupture of coronary aneurysms that can develop during active disease. **B)** Systemic Lupus Erythematosus wouldn't present with a red and swollen tongue or cracked lips. **C)** Kukuchi Fujimoto's is characterized by fevers and cervical lymphadenopathy, not axillary lymphadenopathy, and usually presents in Asian adults. **D)** Multicentric Castleman disease presents with diffuse lymphadenopathy and fevers; it does not present with tongue swelling or cracked lips.

40. **D.** All of the medications listed work very well for rheumatoid arthritis, but methotrexate is in the category of DMARD therapy, which should be utilized first as long as there are no contraindications, such as kidney disease. In the majority of cases, methotrexate will not be enough to control disease and additional medications will need to be implemented such as adalimumab; but a DMARD such as methotrexate is still the first-line therapy.

41. **D.** One of the major goals of therapy in a patient with lupus who is pregnant is to try and keep the disease under control as much as possible. If patients with lupus flare during pregnancy, there is a much higher chance of poor fetal outcomes. Another major consideration is to keep the patient from flaring with the least toxic medications as possible. We know hydroxychloroquine is safe to use during pregnancy, and this medication should always be continued. **B)** Azathioprine is also safe during

pregnancy, but it doesn't sound like the patient needs additional therapy considering her disease is overall stable. If she were having mild flares, then the addition of azathioprine or low-dose prednisone would be reasonable. **C)** Mycophenolate mofetil is contraindicated during pregnancy and should always be avoided in use as it's a known teratogen. **A)** Aspirin use is encouraged along with additional anti-coagulation in pregnant lupus patients who also have anti-phospholipid antibody syndrome. This patient does not have anti-phospholipid antibody syndrome, so she does not need to start aspirin therapy.

42. **B.** Rituximab is a medication that depletes B cells and is a potent immunosuppressive medication. It's also used in the treatment of several malignancies. **A)** Abatacept is a medication that targets T cells and is primarily used in treating rheumatoid arthritis. **C)** Tofacitinib is a medication that blocks multiple cytokine signals through the JAK/STAT system. **D)** Tocilizumab works by blocking interleukin-6.

43. **A.** Out of all of the listed medications, tocilizumab is contraindicated to use in patients with a history of diverticulitis. Any medication that disrupts interleukin-6 signaling should be avoided if possible in patients with a history of diverticulitis as there is an increased risk of bowel perforation in this population. Interleukin-6 likely plays a role in intestinal repair, so blocking this in a patient who already had known intestinal damage increases the risk of bowel perforation. Of note, patients with diverticulosis are still okay to receive the medication. It's only contraindicated if there has been a history of infection of the diverticulosis, which is diverticulitis.

44. **D.** Colchicine is the medication listed that can be used to treat acute gout. Colchicine can be given when a patient has an acute attack as long as the patient has normal kidney function. Another two medication options for treatment of an acute attack are glucocorticoids, such as prednisone, or interleukin-1 inhibition, such as anakinra. **A)** and **B)** Allopurinol and febuxostat are both examples of long-term management of gout and would not help treat an acute gout flare. **C)** Methotrexate is an immunosuppressant medication not used in the treatment of acute or chronic gout.

# Index

**A**

abatacept 15, 18
achilles enthesitis 29
acute lymphoblastic leukemia 104
acute phase proteins 114
adalimumab 14
adaptive immune system 10
adult onset Still's disease 57
alkylating agent 14
allopurinol 43
alprostadil 79
ALPS 99-100
amyloidosis 58
ANA 36, 113
anakinra 15, 43
ANCA antibodies 113
ANCA-associated vasculitis 14, 85, 116
ankylosing spondylitis 25
anti-beta-2 glycoprotein 37
anti-cardiolipin 37
anti-CCP 114
anti-centromere antibody 77-8, 113
anti-chromatin antibody 36, 112-3
anti-cyclic citrullinated peptide (CCP) 22, 114
anti-double-stranded DNA antibody 112
Anti-DS-DNA 113
anti-histone antibody 37, 112-3
Anti-Jo-1 113
anti-malarial drugs 12
anti-nuclear antibodies 111
anti-phospholipid antibody syndrome 116
anti-ribonucleoprotein (RNP) antibody 36, 112-13
Anti-SCL70 (topoisomerase) antibody 77
anti-Smith antibody 36, 112-13
anti-SSA/SSB antibody 36, 72-3112-13
anti-streptolysin O test 50
antiphospholipid syndrome 37
antisynthetase antibodies 113
antisynthetase syndrome 95
AOSD 57
apremilast 17
Arcalyst 15
arthrocentesis 6, 8
ASO 50
auto-antibodies 111
autoimmune eye disease 100
autoimmune hepatitis 112
autoimmune inflammatory joint 3

autoimmune juvenile idiopathic arthritis 106
autoimmune lymphoproliferative syndrome 100
autoimmune pancreatitis 99
autoinflammatory disease 56
azathioprine 13, 80

**B**

B cells 10
B-cell depleting therapy 16
B-cell lymphoma in Sjögren's 72
BAFF factor 16
Behcet's disease 84
belimumab 16-8, 38
biphosphonates 103
BLyS factor 16
bone mineral density 103
Bouchard node 4
birefringence, 41, 42
butterfly rash 34

**C**

C-ANCA 88, 113
C-reactive protein 114
calcium pyrophosphate dehydrate 43
canakinumab 15
CAPS 59
carpometacarpal joint 4
Castleman disease 99
CCP 22
CD20 receptor 16
Cellcept 13-4, 38
central nervous system vasculitis 84
central pain 3
certolizumab pegol 14
chikungunya 53
chlamydia 26
chondrocalcinosis 65
chondrocalcinosis of triangular fibrocartilage 44
chondromalacia patella 108
Churg-Strauss syndrome 87
Cimzia 14
CMC 4
Cogan syndrome 101
colchicine 17, 43
COX-1 11
COX-2 11
CPPD 43
Crohn's disease 26
crowned dens 45
cryoglobulinemic vasculitis 89

cryoglobulins 89
cryopyrin-associated periodic syndromes 59
crystalline arthritis 3-4, 40
Cushingoid appearance 12
cyclophosphamide 14, 18, 38
cytokine 9
cytotoxic T cells 10

**D**

dactylitis 26
dapsone 17
denosumab 103
dermatomyositis 91
diffuse alveolar hemorrhage 36
diffuse infiltrative lymphocytosis syndrome 100
diffuse scleroderma 77
DILS 99-100
DIPs 4
Disease-Modifying Anti-Rheumatic Drugs 12
distal interphalangeal joints 4
DMARDs 12, 18, 31, 108
double stranded DNA 36-7
drug-induced lupus 37
DS-DNA 112
dual energy x-ray absorptiometry 103

**E**

effusion 7
EGPA 15
ELISA 113
Enbrel 14
enthesitis-related juvenile idiopathic arthritis 108
eosinophilic fasciitis 79
eosinophilic granulomatosis with polyangiitis 15, 87
erythema marginatum 41, 49
erythema nodosum 98
erythrocyte sedimentation rate 114
ESR 114
etanercept 14
Ewing sarcoma 105

**F**

familial cold autoinflammatory syndrome 59
familial mediterranean fever 15, 58
febuxostat 43
Felty's syndrome 22
fibromyalgia 3, 67

Forteo 103
full house histology in lupus 35

**G**
giant cell arteritis 80
glucocorticoids 11-2
golimumab 14
gonococcal arthritis 6, 48, 54, 107
gonorrhea 48
Goodpasture's disease 87
gout 4, 40
granulomatosis with polyangiitis
    85, 99

**H**
Hashimoto's thyroiditis 111-12
Heberden's nodes 4
helper T-cells 10
hemochromatosis 65
hemophagocytic lymphohistiocytosis 57
Henoch- Schönlein-purpura 109
hepatitis B 53
hepatitis C 53
HIV 53
HLA-B27 30
HLH 57
HMG-COA reductase 92
Humira 14
hydralazine 37, 112
hydroxychloroquine 13, 38
hyperimmunoglobulin D syndrome 59

**I**
IBD-associated arthritis 26
IgA vasculitis 109
IgG4-related disease 98
IL inhibitors 14, 17
IL-17 11
IL-5 11, 18
IL-6 15
Ilaris 15
immune system 9
immune thrombocytopenic purpura 34
Imuran 13
inclusion body myositis 95
indirect immunofluorescence assay 111
infection-induced ANCA 89
infectious arthritis 3
infective endocarditis 48
inflammatory arthritis 2, 19
inflammatory bowel disease associated
    arthritis 25-6
inflammatory joint pain 2
inflammatory markers 114
inflammatory myopathies 91, 112 116
infliximab 14
innate immune system 9
interleukin 9
interleukin inhibitors 14

interleukin-1 inhibitors 15, 18
interleukin-12 15
interleukin-12/23 inhibitor 17-8
interleukin-17 15, 17-8
interleukin-23 15
interleukin-5 15, 17-8
interleukin-6 15, 17-8
interstitial lung disease 36
interstitial lung disease in
    scleroderma 78
intravenous immunoglobulin 16
isoniazid 112
IVIG 16

**J**
Jaccoud arthropathy 34
JAK/STAT inhibitors 16-8
Janeway lesions 48
JIA 105
joint fluid 5, 7-8
juvenile inflammatory arthritis 105

**K**
Kawasaki disease 110
Kineret 15
knee effusion 7
Kukuchi Fujimoto disease 99-100

**L**
leflunomide 13-4
Legg-Calve-Perthes disease 108
lesinurad 43
Libman-Sacks endocarditis 36
limited scleroderma 76
Löfgren syndrome 98
lupus 23
lupus anticoagulant 37
lupus nephritis 34
lupus overlap syndromes 38
Lyme disease 51, 107

**M**
macrophage activation syndrome 57, 61
malar rash 34-5
MCPs 3
mechanic's hands 95
mediterranean fever 58
mepolizumab 15
metabolic myopathies 94
metacarpophalangeal joints 3
methotrexate 13, 38
microangiopathic hemolytic anemia 78
microscopic polyangiitis 87
migratory arthritis 5
migratory inflammatory arthritis 48
minocycline 37, 112
mixed connective tissue disease 38, 95
monoarticular arthritis 4
moon facies 12

morphea 78
MPO 88
MRI 7
Muckle-Wells syndrome 59
muscular dystrophies 94
musculoskeletal arthritis 3
mycophenolate mofetil 13, 38

**N**
nail fold capillaroscopy 76
nail pitting 28
necrotizing myopathy 91
neonatal-onset multisystem
    inflammatory disease 59
nephrogenic systemic fibrosis 78
neuroblastoma 104
NOMID 59
non-inflammatory arthritis 4, 62
non-inflammatory joint pain 2, 3
non-migratory arthritis
non-steroidal anti-inflammatory drugs 11
nontuberculosis mycobacterium 50
NSAIDs 11
Nucala 15

**O**
oculofacial-skeletal myorhythmia 52
oligoarticular arthritis 6
oligoarticular juvenile idiopathic
    arthritis 107
OMM 52
Orencia 15
Osgood-Schlatter disease 108
Osler's nodes 48
osteoarthritis 3, 4, 63
osteopenia 103
osteopenia, in RA 23
osteophytes 65
osteoporosis 103
osteosarcoma 104
Otezla 17
overlap syndrome 113

**P**
P-ANCA 88, 113
palindromic rheumatoid arthritis 24
panniculitis 98
parathyroid hormone 103
parvovirus B19 52
pauci-immune histology 35
pediatric rheumatology 103
pediatric vasculitis 109
pegloticase 43
pencil-in-cup changes 30-1
pentoxifylline 79
periodic fever 56
peripheral SpA 26
PGE4 inhibitor 18
PIPs 3

Plaquenil 13, 38
polarized microscopy 41
polyarteritis nodosa 83
polyarticular arthritis 6
polyarticular juvenile idiopathic
    arthritis
polymyalgia rheumatica 81
polymyositis 38, 91
PR3 88
probenecid 43
procainamide 112
progressive mulifocal
    leukoencephalopathy 16
Prolia 103
propylthiouracil 112
proximal interphalangeal joints 3
pseudo-meningitis 45
pseudo-rheumatoid arthritis 44
pseudogout 4, 43, 65
psoriatic arthritis 4, 25-6, 28, 108
pulmonary hypertension 36
pulmonary hypertension in
    scleroderma 78

**R**
rapid strep antigen detection test 50
Raynaud's phenomenon 75
reactive arthritis 25-6, 107
Reiter's syndrome 25
relapsing polychondritis 102
Remicade 14
renal tubular acidosis in Sjögren's 72
retroperitoneal fibrosis 99
reversible cerebral vasoconstriction
    syndrome 84
rheumatic fever 49
rheumatoid arthritis 2, 4, 20, 112, 114
rheumatoid factor (RF) 22, 114
rheumatoid factor positive polyarticular
    disease 107
rheumatoid nodules 22
rifampin 112
rilonacept 15
rituximab 16-8
RNA polymerase III 77-8
RNA polymerase III antibody 113

Ro/LA 112
Ross river virus 54
RS3PE 24

**S**
saddle nose deformity 86, 102
sarcoidosis 97, 107
Schirmer's test 73
schistocytes 78
Schober test 29
sclerodactyly 76
scleroderma 38, 75, 112-13, 116
scleroderma renal crisis 78
septic arthritis 105
septic joint 8, 47
seronegative rheumatoid arthritis 22
seropositive rheumatoid arthritis 22
serpiginous rash 49
shrinking lung syndrome 36
sialometry 73
sildenafil in scleroderma 79
Simponi 14
Sjögren's syndrome 71, 116
SLE 23
slipped capital femoral epiphysis 108
spondyloarthritis (SpA) 2, 4, 25,
    28, 107
squaring of the CMC 4
Stelara 15
steroid 11
strawberry tongue 110
subchondral cysts 65
subchondral sclerosis 65
sulfasalazine 13
Susac disease 101
swan neck deformity 21
Sydenham's chorea 49
syndesmophyte 30
synovitis 6
systemic juvenile idiopathic arthritis 106
systemic lupus erythematosus 2, 33, 38,
    107, 112, 116

**T**
T cell interference 15, 17-8
T cells 10

T-score 103
Takayasu's arteritis 82
targeted therapy 14, 17
telangectasias in scleroderma 76
temporal arteritis 80
tenosynovitis 28
tenosynovitis in gonorrhea 49
teriparatide 103
Th1 cell 10
TH2 cell 10
TNF 9
TNF inhibitors 14, 17-8, 112
TNF-alpha 11
TNFRSF1A gene 58
TNG-gamma 11
tofacitinib 16
tophi 41
topoisomerase 77
transverse myelitis 36
TRAPS 58
triangular fibrocartilage 44
tuberculosis 50
tumor necrosis factor 9
tumor necrosis factor receptor-1 58
tumor-necrosis factor inhibitors 14

**U**
ulcerative colitis 2
ulnar deviation of fingers 22
ultrasound 7
uric acid 41
ustekinumab 15
uveitis/conjunctivitis in SpA 28

**V**
vasculitis 80
Viagra in scleroderma 79
Vogt-Koyanagi-Harada disease 101

**W**
Wegener's disease 85
Whipple's disease 52

**X**
x-rays 7
Xeljanz 16